THE HOSPITAL OF MAKE-BELIEVE: FIRST FLOOR

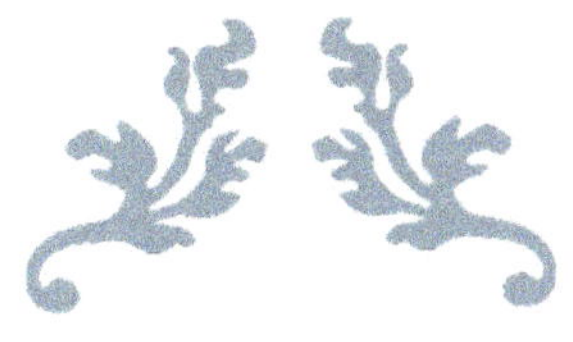

THE HOSPITAL OF MAKE-BELIEVE: FIRST FLOOR

Written by: Kris Stegall, MSN, RN, CEN, MOM

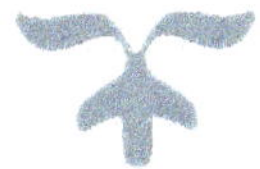

XULON PRESS

Xulon Press
555 Winderley Pl, Suite 225
Maitland, FL 32751
407.339.4217
www.xulonpress.com

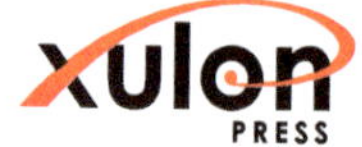

Paperback ISBN-13: 979-8-86850-608-6
Ebook ISBN-13: 979-8-86850-609-3

Dedication

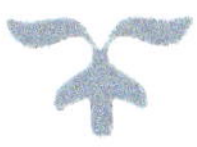

I've been a nurse for over forty years, but two people have indelibly shaped my nursing career. I wish I could introduce you to both.

Michael "The Situation" Tucker, an honored police officer, taught me more about patience under fire, kindness to strangers, and never giving up. Michael had a rare cancer that slowly overtook his life but never dampened his zest for living. Twice he beat the cancer back to return to duty. He influenced the kind of nurse I want to become. I want to be that nurse who stands beside you on your worst day, just to watch you either walk on water or grow wings and fly away. With Miss Anita's blessing (Michael's Mom), I credit Michael with the inspiration to share my stories . . . he is truly my hero!

I wish you could meet the best nurse I ever worked with, Laura Archbald, RN, extraordinaire. We began our trauma nursing career together, raised families, and survived divorces. We each went on to marry the man of our dreams! She taught me that humor is critical to survival and showed me how to see past the sadness of the moment. She kept me safe in my early years as an ER nurse. I watched her talk a man out of a gun in a parking lot, drag me to safety when a patient threw a stretcher at us, keep me calm when my sister died, grab the keys out of a truck that drove into the ER waiting room and take the blame for dressing up a resident for a

Halloween contest at a local establishment, near the hospital (Won first place!). Her guiding air of calmness during utter chaos made survival-mode doable. I watched as she refused ridiculous orders by feigning a hearing problem until the doctor got it right. Her quick thinking rubbed off on me. I miss her every day.

Kris Stegall, RN MSN CEN TNCC MOM

The Hospital of Make-Believe

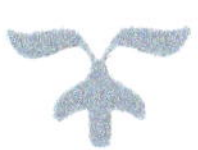

Chapters:

1

The Heart of a Nurse

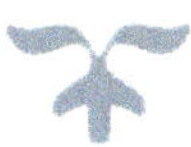

It was a shift change, and the nurse was checking her rooms for the first time. In the first room, a young girl, known for recurrent alcohol withdrawals, was sullen and silent. Her mother stood, tears falling at the bedside. Now was not the time to speak, so the nurse completed her job and walked into the next room. She stood there as a physician had to tell an older man and his family that he had multiple cancer sites in his back and possibly his lymph nodes. "My life is over," said the patient. The doctor left. The nurse countered with, "Nope, not today! Today, you make no decisions except to tell this problem who is the boss . . . you either boss it down or let it run your life." His wife took his hand and nodded . . . a small nervous smile escaped her lips. The nurse left to answer another patient's light. It was the young girl. Her eyes were swollen from crying. The nurse touched her patient's tear-stained cheek and asked, "You think your life is over?" The girl nodded. The nurse whispered, "You have a second chance to make this right. I just left a patient who is all out of second chances. Make the most of this one. Don't waste time feeling sorry for yourself. Be the boss of you!" The nurse reached for the girl's hand, and Mom walked back into the room and asked, "Did I miss something?" "No," replied the nurse. "Just making sure we covered all the bases before admission." She looked back at the young woman, and for the first time, there was the hint of a smile, followed by, "I think I've got this." The nurse smiled and said, " I believe you do," and walked out to answer the next patient light. Sometimes life is just figuring out who the boss of you really is.

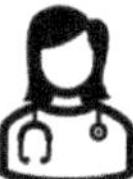

God created the world in seven days. He had already experienced lies, unfaithfulness, and loneliness, but He believed that there was an outside chance for the world to still succeed . . . so He created a nurse.

At first, the heart of nurses was found in mothers, midwives, elders, and volunteers. It was seen in war, on battlefields, and during pandemics. God watched the progress. He knew we would need someone with exceptional skills, a heart that would break over the circumstances of others but never sit in judgment; hands that would hold others when their world fell apart, and a spirit that could welcome new life in one moment and stand with those whose time to die had come the next, doing both with a reassuring spirit . . . so He created a nurse.

He needed someone to walk into the dirtiest place the world has to offer and know how to clean it with hard work and caring so that the next patient has a safe place to begin their journey. There would be double shifts and sometimes weeks with much prayer and little sleep. He needed someone to pick up the collective pieces and create a positive journey for the runaway, the sexually abused woman, the culturally unacceptable man, the angry child, the soldier with the blank stare, the prisoner, the grandfather without any family present, and the quiet, but troubled youth . . . so He created a nurse.

By expecting much and promising little, God directed the passionate heart of one with the gift of healing a wounded soul, advocating for others, and never shying away from a battle. So, He created a nurse.

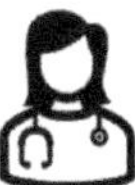

It's not in our nature to give up being an advocate for those who are not up to the task but put up a convincing smoke screen so they will be left alone. Trying to intimidate me doesn't help you get what you want, either. Try being truthful. I understand you are a veteran. I get that your family has given up on you. You've run out of places to hide. No one will fill your prescriptions. Help Lines may put you on hold. Your tall tales fall on deaf ears. You're running out of options. Know that ER nurses listen, Paramedics listen, Police and Fire personnel listen . . . we want to help . . . but you must give up part of your panicked control. If you become aggressive, so will we, but we will fight to get you the care you need . . . you just don't know if you can trust us yet. We care. You saw me steal your phone for a moment, so I could put the emergency help numbers you or your wife might need on speed dial. The third-speed dial number is mine. Some of us have been in your shoes. Don't give up; it's not in your nature or ours to be quitters.

2

If I had only known…

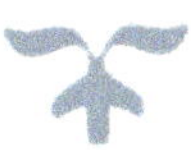

There were two choices, live or die. She entered the ER struggling to stand, held up by two police officers. They headed straight for room #1, the "holding tank" for patients who might try to hurt themselves. The senior officer had done a quick pat down before he put the handcuffs on her, but those were getting ready to come off. The new patient was the poster child for drug abuse. Dirty hair, torn fishnet hose, and chunky high heels. A shower would help immensely. This very sad lady was my next project. I introduced myself and reached out to pat her shoulder. If I can touch people, I can usually control the situation. Those who shrink away are too volatile for me to handle by myself. My patient's name was Gwen, and she spoke softly over a sore and bleeding lip. She looked like she'd been in a fight.

"Could you use a nice hot shower and some clean clothes?" I asked.

"Probably make me wear one of those crazy gowns again," she replied, not making eye contact.

"If you cooperate, I have a set of soft scrubs that you can put on, but you'd have to trust me, and I'll take you to the showers and back." She looked at me with a street cynical glare but then stood up and allowed me to take her arm. I grabbed three fluffy white hospital towels and a patient care kit from a nearby cart. The kit had soap, a toothbrush, mouthwash, shampoo, and a comb. She knew I had to stay while she showered but became sarcastic.

"This how you get your kicks?" she said.

I never rise to the bait, so I replied, "No. This is how I help people to feel a little more human." Gwen stood under the water for almost ten minutes, crying softly, letting tears and warm water run down her face, until I told her we needed to go back. She toweled off and put on the scrub top and bottoms. She seemed calmer, and we walked back to her room. The blank look on her face said the invisible protective barrier was immediately back in place. "Hungry?" I asked.

"No," came the reply a little too quickly. "Where am I supposed to sit?" The room had no furniture for a reason.

The nurse looked around. "I can drag a stretcher pad or a bean bag chair in here."

"Bean bag," said Gwen. So, I put the bag on the floor, left Gwen to her own thoughts, and made rounds on other patients. My gut feeling was that Gwen had suffered some deep abuse and was trying to cover the scars by drinking and taking any pills she could find. No one came with her or called to check on her, so she was totally alone. On my next pass by #1, I grabbed my lunch and two juice drinks and went into Gwen's room. She looked startled when I dragged a second bean bag in to sit on.

"What are doing? Are you the shrink now too?" She looked genuinely surprised.

"Nope, I'm just the nurse who never gets to eat my lunch, so I thought I'd share it with you." She looked suspicious, but who could resist my homemade chicken salad sandwich? I held out a partially wrapped half and pushed a drink at her.

"Do they let you do this?" she said as she bit into her sandwich.

"Nope, but not enough to stop me." Gwen smirked. I smiled . . . a smart aleck lived inside Gwen, and I could respect that. "So, what's your story?"

"Why?" she asked and took a long drink of her juice. "What's in it for me?"

"If you'll tell me your story, then I can tell you what your options are." She again looked suspicious but began to tell me of a life filled with abuse. There was physical and sexual abuse from close family members since age seven. First, she stole her mother's medications, and then she traded sex for drugs. Her father died last summer from cancer, her mother refuses to speak to her, and in halting tones, she told me about her daughter, who she hadn't seen in two years. Her eyes filled with tears.

"I'm just a horrible person. Who would want to be around me?"

"I would," I said, looking her steadily in the eye. She looked away and shook her head. "You don't understand."

"OK, then make me understand. Do you think you are the only one who has 'scars' from life? Go for it. Give me the list." So, Gwen did.

"I'm depressed and have thought about just taking my life."

"Do you have a plan?" I asked, hoping that she didn't have a current one.

"No, but it's the easy way out," she said.

"Well, I've been there," I volunteered, "but it's a choice . . . go on."

"My father sexually abused me when I was little. That's why I left home."

This was said to try to shock me, but I replied, "I've been there and got the tee-shirt." Keep going.

"My family doesn't care anymore, and they don't speak to me or help me out." She punctuated the sentence by spitting on the floor, but not near me.

"Well, I have one of those families, too," I sighed. "What else?"

She looked at me quizzically, "and I have been in jail for drugs, and I hate my life."

"Is that it?" I asked, cleaning up the papers from our meal.

"So, what if it is? What are you gonna do about it?" She almost used the words as a sword to jab me.

"Well, except for the jail time, I can match you blow for blow, and a lot of your life is like mine. We all have scars, but I'm standing here today, happy and in control of my life." I let that sink in. "So, my question to you is 'Live or Die'?"

"That's it? That's your plan?" That's all you got?" Gwen looked stunned.

"Yup . . . live or die . . . pick one. I don't have all night here," I added.

Gwen looked shocked and asked, "What happens if I pick die?"

"Well, then I feed and water you, give you a nice warm blankie, and you get some much-needed sleep. Eventually, you get a room, and I go back to caring for my other patients."

"But what if I pick live?" she asked slowly.

"Then you make a choice to survive, and we make a plan that starts today. I have most of the scars you have, and I have walked that path. I will share my survival with you and find you a place to live as long as you keep trying and don't give up."

Gwen looked shocked. "What if I fall down? Then what? You give up on me?"

I put my arm around her and said, "No, I give you a hand to get back up. If you want to try, I will help you."

She thought about it for a long minute. "How did you 'get out' from your abuse when you were little?"

"I talked to my pastor, hid in my closet, got counseling, and figured out that none of this was my fault. I deserved better, and so do you. You can earn your right back to be respected."

"So, if I pick die?"

"Then I will cover you up and let you be. It's a waste of my time to try and help if it doesn't matter to you."

"But it does . . . I mean, I want it to matter . . . I pick 'live.'" Gwen's tears fell as she grabbed my hand.

"OK, we will start in the morning," I said.

"But I have no place to stay . . . I've been thrown out," she sobbed. I hugged her.

"Let me work on that," I said. "Get some rest. You're gonna need it." So, Gwen lay down and slept until about 6:00 a.m. Breakfast arrived, and she ate it. "Feeling a bit better" I asked? Gwen looked rough but was hanging in there. "I found you a room at the Good Will Enterprise's. They will help you with clothing, food, and counseling. You'll be near a bus line, so you can get a job. If you use drugs, you're out. If you become argumentative, you're out. If you give up . . . you're out. So, what will it be?"

"I'm in," said Gwen. I dropped Gwen off at Goodwill on my way home, and it was about three weeks later, she came back to the ER with a sprained ankle. She had a job as a cashier at Walmart but had fallen and injured her foot. When I asked her what else was up, she showed me applications for a local art school. She wanted a scholarship. My heart skipped a beat . . . Gwen was serious about choosing "Live." So, we shared my lunch again, and I helped her fill out the applications. As it turns out, Gwen was quite a talented lady and managed to win a scholarship that paid for her first year. My fellow ER Peeps pooled their pocket money and gave Gwen enough McDonald's certificates that she wouldn't be hungry for six months! She was looking for a roommate and said she was going to Alcoholics Anonymous. She shyly showed me her first 30-day chip for being sober. I hugged her and so did several staff members. She beat the odds . . . hopefully, she was on a good life roll. Grace was leaving but turned to ask me, "What made the difference for you? How did you get past all the awful things?"

"I took the hand up when it was offered. I refused to feel sorry for myself. I fell down a lot, but I realized it's only failure if you don't get back up. Now it's a way of life that you pay forward."

Gwen teared up but quickly wiped them away. She smiled and said, "I pick 'Live' every day I wake up . . . thank you." And she was gone. On the stretcher was one McDonald's certificate with three words written on it: "I Pick Live." I held the paper and put it in my pocket. I tried to wipe away the tears as I turned to go into the next patient room. Today was "Best Day Ever!"

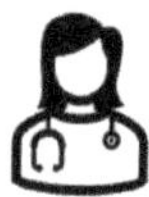

I hate returning phone calls to patients I know nothing about, but I seem to spend a lot of time doing that. I had to call a fifteen-year-old girl about a positive pregnancy test, but legally, her father had a right to know. Of course, he answered the phone.

Nurse: May I speak to Andrea?

Dad: This is her dad. You can tell me the test results.

Nurse: "Do you and your daughter talk much?"

Dad: "Yes . . . I know she's pregnant. I just need the numbers from the test so I can make an appointment for her to see my wife's doctor. It's been about ten years since I had to deal with this.

Nurse: "OK, write this down." She gives the results. "Sir, may I ask you a question?"

Dad: "Sure . . . what is it?"

Nurse: "You seem pretty calm . . . how does that work?"

Dad: "Of course, I'm sad this came up this way . . . but it's a baby, and they don't know they weren't expected. It's like if the Queen of

England just showed up at your house; you'd invite her in. It's just what families do."

Nurse: "and . . ."

Dad: "She's my daughter . . . who else is going to love her like I can?"

Nurse: "It's been such a long day, sir . . . but you've just made mine."

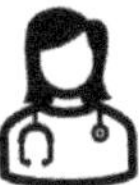

Pain means different things to different people. Working as a Head Nurse for an Adventure Race, I see so many unusual things that I have learned to let them "play out" if they are not life-threatening. My husband is a Paramedic and has a unique command of the 0-10 Pain Scale.

A middle-aged female participant injured her arm at the finish line. My husband, a medic, was called to evaluate the patient. She was alert, standing up, breathing, and holding her injured arm close to her body.

Paramedic: "How bad is your pain on the 0-10 scale?"

Injured Runner: **"A *TEN*"** she says, as all the people around her nod with great understanding.

Paramedic: "If it's a 10, I will have you transported immediately. If it was, say, a 4–5, you could probably get your beer and tee shirt first before you mosey over to the medical tent." The injured woman thinks about it for a couple of seconds. Her friends are all drinking beer.

Injured Runner: "It's just a 3 or maybe a 3 1/2. I'll be over in a few minutes."

The Paramedic walks back to the medical tent and waits. In about ten minutes, the injured party, accompanied by three friends, shows up with a beer and tee shirt. She has a minimally fractured arm, is splinted, and is sent on her way. I wouldn't have believed it, if I hadn't watched the story play out. Pain is relative to what your priorities are.

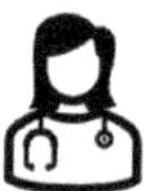

I get $1 extra an hour to be the charge nurse, but that is not the reason I do it. I'm taking one for the team and hoping we all survive the night. There are nights when you are in charge, and you simply take whatever is tossed to you. Then there are those nights when you think you have no well-thought-out plan . . . and God throws you a great curve. It is impossible to please all the families . . . and there are times when staff contributes to making things worse. Imagine a family who tells the nurse that they will only complete treatment when their mom arrives. They are old enough to sign up for care but suddenly are acting like children. You smile, sweat, and wonder how you can make this sad experience more positive and still deliver good care. The family isn't being unreasonable, but there is a visible strain on everyone's faces. Staff has basically washed their hands and backed off to a safe distance. They call me to the lobby . . . MOM is here. Great, this night can only get worse. I go out thinking, "I'll figure this out as I go," and then I see her. She just happens to be one of my dearest work friends. I've never met her family . . . and now I have. What a great treat in an evening when anxiety ran so high! It was like a cold, clean breath of fresh air. It's rare to get a second chance to make it right . . . but at least on one night, I did. Imagine the faces of the staff when we came back to the room doing the "Tootsie Roll" walk together!

3
What do I do now?

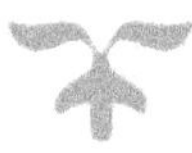

Funerals are hard. I haven't been to very many patient services in my nursing lifetime, but this young man made a permanent mark on my heart. Today, we celebrated Officer Michael Darnell "The Situation" Tucker Jr. He was both a father and a hero. With his permission, he has "graced" *The Hospital of Make-Believe* with his humor, caring, and warrior spirit to overcome cancer twice. We said goodbye today. As police officers from Maryland, Washington DC, and Virginia, one mayor, a police chief, and many healthcare workers, family, and friends gathered, we gave him a warrior's send-off. I was overwhelmed by the multicultural gathering of professionals and family . . . but not more than when a wonderful Environmental Service friend sitting near me began showing me videos on her phone of Michael laughing and kidding with her while she cleaned his hospital room. I think everyone he met was touched by his wonderful spirit . . . and then there was always that "man" cologne he wore, the Cool Water and Chrome. No one wore it better. The Town of Seat Pleasant's Police Chief, Christopher Portillo, announced that their new helicopter will be named after the officer who made a difference in the lives of those he served. His call sign, "Tucker" will soon be airborne and still watching over his charges. I invite you to know the man we honor. Here is my favorite picture of Michael Tucker. He is unforgettable.

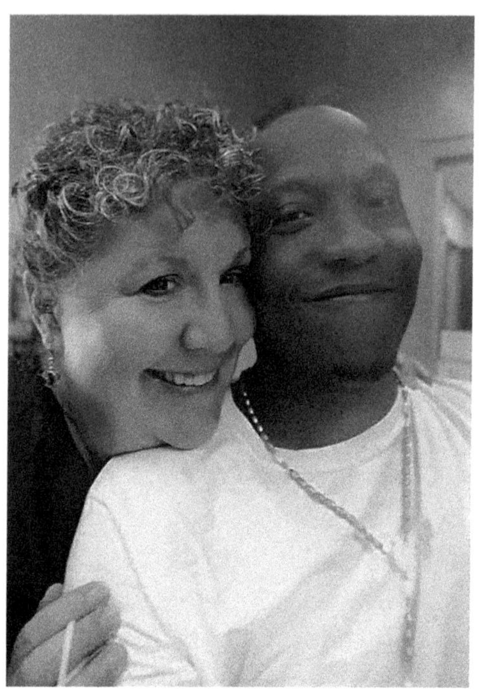

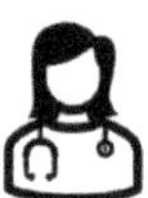

Sometimes, words are just not enough, and I struggle just to listen. I went into a room to answer a light, and a fragile older woman needed a bedpan. Her family had gone, and I helped her. I tipped the stretcher with the feet down to allow gravity to help the process, and she laughed. When everything was done, I asked her how long she'd been fighting her battle with cancer . . . the headscarf and bruised arms were a giveaway. She smiled and told me her story, but then she asked me why all her "friends" never talked to her anymore and wondered aloud why I was being so bold? I sat beside her and said, "Because they are afraid they will say the wrong thing or that you don't want company." She said, "I miss them . . . what can I do?" So, I shared with her my journey of miscarriages and a stillbirth. Initially, my answering machine was my best friend. Then visitors, who were tired of my not returning their calls, showed up in person, unannounced. My church family kept mis-stepping. First, they came in a group to my house and brought me a "baby feet" pin; the kind you give women who have had an abortion. I knew they misunderstood what it meant, but it still hurt my feelings. On the occasion I tried to come back to church, they ambushed me with "I'm sorry" and quoted Bible verses. The worst was, "To all things, there is a season." At that point, all I wanted to do was punch them in the mouth, but I settled for running into the restroom . . . sadly, it was the men's room. The nice gentleman who was washing his hands had no idea why this "ugly crying" woman was standing beside him, but to his credit, he announced, "I'll stand guard outside until you're done." At that moment, I loved him because he didn't require an explanation. So here is what I learned, and I shared it with my sweet patient.

1) Throw a bunch of towels or sheets in a clothes basket and pour coffee/soda on them. When someone asks what they can do for you, produce the laundry. Ask them to bring it back at an agreed-upon time (when you would like some company) and tell them how you want it folded. They will have a mission, and you will have company when you're ready. And who doesn't like clean towels?

2) Keep a list of things people can do for you. Wash your car, mow your lawn, bring some fresh daisies, fix brown bag snacks for your kids, bring apple juice or your favorite bottled water, fix a single-serve meal in a disposable pan (nothing is worse than enough Lasagna for a week), sweep your front porch, and keep a short grocery list of things that do not require refrigeration so they can be left on your porch.

3) When you're ready to venture into the world, take a loud friend. After the "men's room" incident, I got my very loud friend,

who wasn't a churchgoer, to escort me to and from church for a few weeks. I needed a "guard," and she needed a church. The first time a group started to tell me how sorry they were for me, I started to tear up; she simply held up her hand like she was parting the Red Sea and screamed, "Get back!" We continued to our seats without so much as a concerned look in our direction. She literally kept me from crying, and we both ended up in hysterics at the back of the church. I came into my own calmness eventually and was able to manage by myself . . . but literally thanked God for her plain-spoken words when I could not find my own. When people do not know what to say, they inevitably say the "wrong" thing (under pressure). Let people know how they can help and encourage them to come by and visit for a few minutes. You might need it as much as they do. I know my patient did.

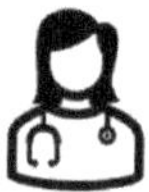

"You most likely have cancer," said the doctor as he was filling out a form on the clipboard. The older couple reached to hold hands, and the nurse stood behind them, watching the drama unfold.

"Is my husband going to die?" asked the wife.

The doctor didn't look up from his paperwork. "He has a few spots on his liver and intestines."

Looking anxious, the wife asked, "How many spots?"

The doctor continued to study his paperwork. "We don't really count them, ma'am"

"So, there are too many to count?" (wife tears up)

The doctor looked toward the door and said, "We'll work on a plan and see how it unfolds." It sounded like something a coach would say to a losing athletic team.

His wife stood up and asked, "Tomorrow? On Sunday, you'll do that?"

In his most doctor sterile voice, the replied, "Most likely on Monday. There are a few more tests to run. My colleague or a consultant will be planning your care," and he left quickly.

The husband exhales loudly and says, "So, nurse . . . don't they work on the weekend around here? I guess I'm old enough to die." He looks at the nurse for approval.

"I'd imagine you could do just about anything . . . but there are no decisions to be made until you get the whole story. I have time right now to give you an idea of what to expect in the next few days (the nurse doesn't have time but makes time). Give me just a minute." (She brings back three popsicles!) "I find that popsicles and warm blankets make most problems a little easier to handle." (Husband and wife smile, blinking back tears and all three begin to eat the popsicles).

The husband looks at his wife of forty-three years, still holding her hand, and says, "I don't know what to do . . ."

His wife smiles finally and says, "You'll do exactly what I tell you to do . . . just like always!" All that could be heard was love and the sound of popsicles.

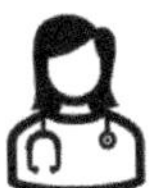

You get a phone call that says the doctor wants you to know you have gonorrhea. The nurse tells you the diagnosis, tells you how to get rid of it, and hangs up. You called back three times, hoping to get someone to explain what that really means to you. You yell into the phone. The nurse gives you the same diagnosis. You think your life is ruined. You blame the nurse . . . you say the doctor is stupid . . . you'll get a second opinion.

The same nurse must call another patient and tell them the X-rays are suspicious of cancer. She looks at them and reads the radiologist's notes. She calls because charging them another copay to get bad news seems wrong. When the news is delivered, there is silence, breath-holding, and then the exhale.

Wife: "What do I do now?"

Nurse: "You take him to your doctor and see the oncologist. You will learn your care options and decide what to do from there. Take a day to think about it. Talk to your doctor, your pastor, and a trusted friend."

Wife: "How long?" and her voice trails off. The nurse is fighting for control.

Nurse: "I'll send your information to your doctors tomorrow. I will leave a message for them."

Wife: "Do you know how long I've been married to him?"

Nurse: (tearing up) "No . . . how long?"

Wife: "Forty-eight years; . . . we were hoping to make fifty."

Nurse: "Never underestimate yourself . . . the human spirit . . . especially two people that love each other."

Wife: "We might not make it through this . . ."

Nurse: "You will . . ."

Wife: "I bet it's hard to call people with this kind of news."

The nurse is completely undone now, holding her head in her hand on the counter. "Let us know how things go or if we can help." A staff member comes up behind her and puts her hand on the nurse's shoulder. The nurse hears the husband, in the background, asking, "What's wrong?" and the wife says, "I have to go now." The nurse hears her tell him he must go to the doctor's office tomorrow. The line hangs up. There are only nine more hours left in the shift.

4

Did I say that?

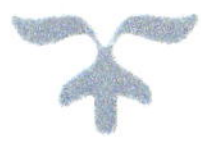

ER nurses have a different way of dealing with behavioral health moments. It's like a safety net to get out alive. The nurse was going through the hourly list of things you ask people who are detoxing. She brushed her patient's hair to try and help her relax. The patient seemed exhausted.

Nurse: "Nausea?"

Patient: "No."

Nurse: "Tremors? Hold your hands out for me. Are you feeling anxious?" Arms extended; she noted the patient's fingers shaking.

Patient: "Yes!"

Nurse: "Visual Hallucinations?"

Patient: "Nope. I don't see things!" She shook her head no for emphasis.

Nurse: Realizing her patient was going to stop answering questions, she said: "Anything bothering you?"

Patient: "Well . . . yes . . . it's those voices."

Nurse: "So, what are they saying to you? Are they happy voices? Sad voices?"

Patient: "NO! They are damned annoying voices. It's like they know it all."

Nurse: "Well, if I heard voices and they annoyed me, I would ignore them. I wouldn't let them be the boss of me anymore." I was sure the Psych floor wouldn't handle things like this, but it was like giving control back to the patient, and that's the important thing, right?

Patient: "You mean act like they aren't there? Like blocking phone calls? I don't have to answer them?"

Nurse: "That's right; it's all up to you," and finished braiding the patient's hair.

Patient: "Wish I'd thought of that sooner. Thanks."

(and for those who were wondering, it worked out fine)

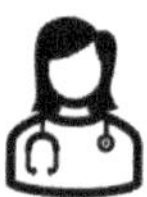

All shift long, a patient had made life difficult for the staff. He screamed obscenities after he pushed the nurse's call light, and someone asked, "if they could help." He threw a cup of coffee at the staff because he didn't get two cups with a meal. He beat his call light into pieces, hammering it on his bedside table. He kept everyone awake, screaming and pushing his bed into the wall repeatedly. It was the overwhelmed third-shift charge nurse who finally stepped up. The patient came out into the hall, threatening staff with verbal abuse, hands clenched, and a fighting posture. The nurse walked up to the patient and surprised him. She stopped, just inside his personal space, and spoke in a low but firm tone. "Do you remember how your Momma used to beat the living daylights out of you for doing something wrong?"

The patient replied sheepishly, "Yeah." The nurse took a quick step toward the patient to close the gap between them. Her staff was concerned, thinking she was going to take a swing and stepped in behind her.

"Well, that's nothing compared to what I'm gonna do if you don't straighten up, shut up, and start realizing that this is not a hotel. GET IN YOUR ROOM NOW!"

The man did an about-face and almost ran back into his room. Later in the shift, when he was seen peeking out his door, a CNA would call out, "She's still here until 7:00 a.m.!" The patient would retreat into his room to watch the clock. When the AM shift came in, they asked how the disgruntled patient was doing and were told, "Fine with us. But if he gets loud, tell him the same Charge Nurse is back tonight."

Sometimes, you just need to communicate clearly in a patient's own language. Do they make translators for that?

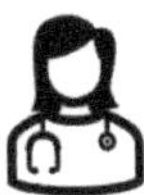

Have you ever been to one of those "be nice" classes where they tell you what not to say? I always get in such trouble there for trying to coach my seatmate into saying nothing and looking straight ahead. They don't want your input, only your obedience to the scripted answers. It's sort of like getting stopped for a traffic violation but admitting to nothing. Maybe if they started out with what you *could* say, it would be easier to swallow. As if you could triage the non-emergent and say, "I realize that it feels like an emergency, but your life is not in danger from vomiting once," OR, "I realize you feel like you are running out of options and up against a deadline of 'tomorrow' to get your sports physical done, but we cannot help you with 'well visits.'" A personal favorite of mine is, "Sorry your car is in the shop, but calling an ambulance for a 'red' finger that hasn't even blistered is not one of the choices anymore. I am sure the spider scared you, but pouring gasoline on him and trying to light a match was a poor choice. I do have a Band-Aid for your boo-boo," and sometimes, I will put an air kiss on it to show that I do care. Some things can be quickly fixed . . . but a lot of things cannot be easily fixed. We need to save our time and resources for those true emergencies. Just take a breath and let the reality sink in. It's like being stuck in traffic and needing to relieve yourself. Sometimes, there is not a good answer. Now, I take a container of bubbles with me so I can blow them out the window and entertain the other drivers. I may try that at work later this week.

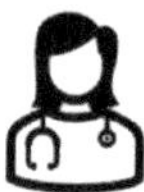

Do you want to create a sensational moment? Try being female and entering the single-seater men's bathroom at an upscale office complex because the women's restroom has an "Out of Order" sign on it. Did I mention I was attending a class training us to be "the best of the best" (yes, more Maverick be nice classes)? The key here is never to wear your name tag. I went in, completed the task, washed my hands, and, for an extra touch, flipped the seat up with the toe of my shoe prior to unlocking the door to leave. A man, probably the same doctor who tried to order me around the day before when I got "misplaced," asked me in that same demanding voice, "Can't you read?" pointing to the Men's Room sign. I smiled my best Nurse smile (as opposed to just stabbing him) and said, "Why yes, I can . . . and you are in luck, sir. I just checked it, and there are no men in there . . . so I left the seat up . . . just for you!." I kept walking to the outside of the building, so he wouldn't know which classroom I was in and waited a moment for him to lock the sacred door, then slid back into my classroom and put my name tag back on.

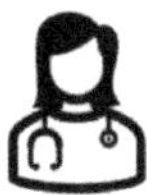

The nurse walks a staff member's family friend out to their car, him on crutches and the nurse carrying bags, shoes, etc. As they reach the car, the patient drops a tissue out of his pocket and reaches for his keys. The patient reaches for the tissue and almost falls off the crutches. The nurse chastises him loudly and kicks the tissue out of the way. He still tries to reach for it, being the gentleman he is, and the nurse slugs him in the shoulder, trying to prevent him from falling. He unlocks the door and sidesteps to move toward the front seat, trying to allow the nurse to move out of the way. He risks falling, and the nurse takes his crutches away as she stuffs him in the driver's seat, despite his protesting. What she saw out of the corner of his eye was another patient leaving the ER. He looked aghast when the nurse slugged the patient and even more put out when she took his crutches away and told him to get in the car! (using very explicit verbiage) She expected to hear a complaint from the "witness" that staff was abusing patients. She called the patient's wife, who said if she ever had to rough him up again, to "just tell 'witnesses' that it was 'my' husband." The nurse smiled. Why hadn't she thought of that?

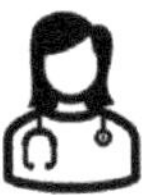

Doctor's offices have established a nursing triage or hotline, as it's known, to try to keep patients from going to the ER for concerns more appropriately handled in an office visit. It's difficult to stop and listen to each concern on the phone, especially if you're busy, but you try . . .

Nurse: "Nurse Hotline (who thought up that catchy line?). Do you have an emergency?"

Caller:" Yeah, I'm having back pain, and it hurts to pee . . . what do you think it is?"

Nurse: "Well, it could be a UTI or cancer. It's hard to tell over the phone. Have you called your Primary Care Provider? They may be able to help."

Caller: "Can you just call something in?"

Nurse: "Like what?"

Caller: "Maybe medicine . . . what do you have?"

Nurse: "I'm all out of miracles, but they do go pretty fast. I do have one or two lottery tickets left . . . ma'am . . . hello?"

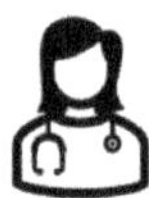

If you are a patient in police custody and decide to fling your dirty underwear in my face because I asked you to provide a urine specimen, know that I will cut your Victoria's Secret panties off and throw them in the red hazmat trash.

Patient: (angry) "Hey! Those were mine!"

Nurse: "*Were*, is the operative word here. They *were* yours. Here, have a pair of our elastic hospital underwear."

Patient: "They don't fit."

Nurse: "I think they are a perfect match for you, ma'am. They are 'safety panties.' If you wear them, you will be "safe."

Patient: (Holds up the elastic mesh, one size fits all panties) "I don't think "safety" means the same thing to you as it does to me."

Nurse: "Maybe not . . . but it isn't my circus, ma'am!"

5

I needed a miracle

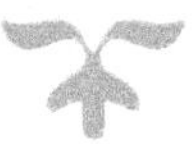

I went to a music concert in Myrtle Beach, South Carolina, years ago with speaker Luis Palau. I generally stay on the fringes of big crowds, but a new friend of mine was scheduled to appear on stage, and I wanted to be supportive. Only 20,000 people showed up, but for the first time, I found myself about four standing rows from center stage. It was honestly a little scary, and back then, no one had cell phones, so I was on my own. I'm watching the crowd and notice a child lying limp in a backpack carrier. Something looked wrong, so I approached him. As I introduced myself to the "parents" as an ER Nurse, the child began to seize actively. The panicked adults answered my rapid-fire questions. They were new foster parents who had picked up the child less than twenty-four hours ago and knew nothing about allergies or medications. I removed the child from the carrier with a kind man's assistance. The seizure passed. I felt for a heartbeat and noted a shallow breathing pattern, but his skin temperature was sky-high. I called for water, and everyone donated their own bottle, which we started pouring over the child. My friend had come out on stage and had already notified Medical of the emergency. Security worked with me to pass the child to the stage where Paramedics received him. He was beginning to wake up, but crowd control and a caring response saved this little boy. Timing is everything, and I have no doubt that God placed me there to help, even though I dislike large crowds. It pays to listen.

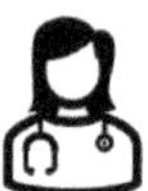

You are probably wondering how nurses have time to meet the perfect companion and find wedded bliss. Sometimes it takes a couple of tries, but as a divorced nurse with a daughter, free time was hard to come by. I didn't go to bars but did fall prey to the "kitchen ladies" at my church, who tried to fix me up with approved young men. I remember walking out of the church with one man, and our only agreement was to have lunch and a good laugh. I was also a charter member of Match.com. I had several failures and was about to give up on dating when I met my beloved Hot Rod. I knew he was the real deal because I recognized his profile picture. Charleston, South Carolina, EMS workers had their ID pictures made at the local jail, and I recognized the background. He was a retired Airborne Ranger working as a Paramedic. For me, it was love at first sight, but we dated to give things an "air of approval" to our kids. On our first date, Rod picked me up after work. We sat for a few moments in his car, deciding where to go eat. Of course, a rather inebriated man came wandering through the street, calling out my name. Jerry was a regular at my ER and was impressed that I appeared to have a car, so he came over and laid on the hood. Rod was not happy with this and started to get out, but I called Jerry over to my open window.

Jerry: "Hi Miss Kris. You got any extra change on ya'? I'm pretty hungry tonight."

Kris: "Jerry, I am going to dinner with this man, and I think he's a keeper. You're ruining our first date!" Rod was being patient and had a slight smile on his face.

Jerry: "Oh (punctuated by horrible breath), I am sooooo sorry, Miss Kris." Then he points at Rod and adds, "She's a really nice lady and she's MY nurse, so you be really good to her." Jerry looked at me for approval, and I nodded.

Kris: (Handing him a snack from her purse) "You come by tomorrow, and I'll let you know how the date went. I bet I can find a sandwich for you too."

Jerry: (Patting the car and straightening up his dirty shirt and jacket) "You kids have a good time! I'll be on my way."

As we watched Jerry stumble off, Rod turned to me and looked very serious.

Rod: "Is this going to happen a lot when we are together? Do you always carry snacks?"

Kris: "Yes, it is, and yes, I do. Why, are you hungry?" I was afraid for a moment that this was the end of our date, but he smiled at me.

Rod: "OK, I can deal with it."

And they lived happily ever after. As a side note on the snacks, I would always pack an extra lunch for Rod because I knew he would toss a brown bag lunch to Johnnie out the window of his ambulance on days he worked near the hospital. Johnnie was our mutual street patient, and Rod looked out for him. How perfect is that?

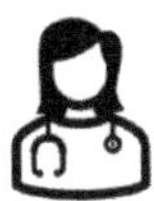

This time it was me. In 2015, I fell down a flight of stairs and sustained a head injury. Thirty days later, I was diagnosed with bilateral subdural hematomas (brain bleeds) and required urgent surgery. My husband was off on a training mission, but I was finally able to reach him, and he was flying in. The staff nurses on the floor were stalling for time so I could see my husband before surgery. Time had run out, and I was being wheeled down the hall. Out of nowhere, my husband appeared, racing down the hall in his BDUs (battle dress uniform) and actually jumped over the stretcher railing to get to me since the transport team was not going to stop (time is money in an OR). He stage whispered to me the words every woman wants to hear when she is afraid she might wake up with permanent brain damage, "Don't worry, Kris. The insurance is all paid up." It was his way of saying everything would be fine; Truly a humor-in-uniform moment. The nursing staff heard it, and when I woke up in the Neuro Intensive Care Unit, social services were asking questions. It seems they were concerned that Rod had pushed me down the stairs to collect the insurance. I survived a slight stroke and was able to return to work in about seven weeks.

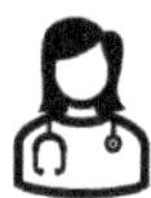

In the summer of 2018, I had an August day off from work, and it had taken about four hours for someone to find me. My phone number had not been updated at my husband's workplace (don't let this happen to you). A friend finally found me, and the news was dire. Rod was near death, lying in a tiny hospital ER near my home. I took off and was at his bedside in about twenty minutes. His team protectively surrounded the stretcher and briefed me on what had happened. Rod had a crushed pelvis, a broken back, and an abdomen full of blood. My ER nurse kicked in, and I had no time to cry. I needed to get him transferred before he bled to death. They wanted paperwork filled out, so I handed it off to a team member. I had the flight team on speed dial, but the weather was bad. I prayed for an immediate solution, and God gave me one. A paramedic tapped me on the shoulder and asked if I remembered him. He was an EMS student I had precepted during his time in the ER. He understood the urgency and offered to take Rod to the nearest Trauma hospital in record time if I could cut through the red tape and get the paperwork done. I walked to the Nursing Station and addressed the entire crew about the transfer. "This place has almost let my husband bleed out and had made no effort to get him to the nearest Interventional Radiology department to fix the immediate problem. I have transport waiting and need you to call 'Trauma 1' with a report." I grabbed up EKGs, radiology reports, and anything else I could get my hands on. While they were packaging Rod up, I stepped up and stage whispered, "I would appreciate it if you would live through this for me." We both deal in deathly humor daily, so this was our norm. His team was leaning in to hear his reply. Through clenched teeth, my Paramedic husband said, "I know why I need to live, but what's your reason?" I told him, "I have become very attached to the Blue Cross insurance. If you could live and work two more years to retirement, we could have it for life. I could also become real attached to that blue handicapped parking sticker we're gonna get. If you don't live, I won't get the best parking!" Rod's answer was, "Roger that." It was about then his team looked at me as they all took a giant step back from the stretcher. They had seen me picking up test results and handed me a handful they had gathered as we left for the Trauma Hospital. His team drove my car, so I could ride with Rod. They were invisible until I needed anything, but one or two men stayed with me 24/7, so I didn't have to listen to doctors tell me it was "touch and go" alone. I was never without food or coffee. They stayed through the multiple surgeries and, since I had no family nearby, made arrangements for me to get some sleep (while someone stayed with Rod) and supplied me with a change of clothes and a toothbrush. When Rod was transferred to the Rehab facility, a hot-spot Wi-Fi and an electric ice chest appeared in his room. His bed was decorated in climbing ropes with carabiners clipped in for good measure, and my spot on the broken couch had a lovely pillow and quilt. Is it any wonder that when the Rehab kicked him out two weeks early for being an over-achiever? His team showed up at my house and built a ramp so I could get Rod's wheelchair inside. I can't show you the picture but imagine them posing as "Charlie's Angels" with saws, axes, and electric drills. It was priceless. These men were my salvation. My initial prayer for a miracle brought me a paramedic to save Rod's life and continued by surrounding me with a team of caring "angels," although they would be quick to say they were just doing their job. Sometimes, family is not who you are born to but is created by those who stick by you. The caring hearts of Rod's team members got us through some scary tough days.

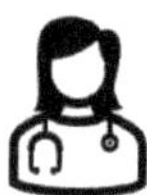

An ER nurse went to start an IV on an older woman who had a heart rate of over 150 beats a minute and needed cardiac medication immediately. Band-Aids on both arms showed evidence of multiple unsuccessful attempts to secure IV access. The nurse introduced herself and placed a warm hand on her cold shoulder. The patient tearfully asked her if she was a specialist, and the nurse said:

Nurse: "I am the IV specialist you need." The patient was refusing an IV in her hand, but there wasn't much choice. "So, can I try to make you feel better?" She began warming the patient's hand by holding it between her hands.

Patient: "Well, OK, I guess you can." There were two nursing students in the room with their instructor, standing silently. The nurse drew a student to the bedside and had her flush an IV connector and hold tape.

Nurse: (Leans over to the patient and whispers loudly at close range) "OK, we can do this, but I need your help. You must hold your mouth just right to make this happen." The distraction took her mind off the needle the nurse was holding.

Patient: "I don't understand what to do!" she said anxiously.

Nurse: "Just do this," and showed her best imitation of Duck Lips. The patient concentrated and tried to purse her lips together correctly. "Thanks, perfect. Hold that pose." The nurse still had her own Duck Lips set in place, and out of the corner of her eye, she noticed the two nursing students showing the patient their best Duck Lips! They were encouraging the patient the best way they could. The instructor stood apart from his students with a frown on his face. The IV was completed in one attempt and taped down. The Nurse supervised the identification, drawing up, and injection of the cardiac medication by the students. The Nursing instructor chose not to participate in the Duck Lips IV placement but told the students that they would present an after-action review (AAR) at the end of their shift. I would have so loved to be a fly on the wall when they showed their classmates the Duck Lips and explained their first emergency treatment. I think those two students will grow up to be awesome nurses!

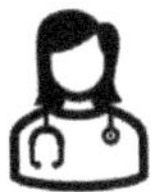

Long ago and far away, try to imagine that you are a dialysis patient, on your way to your doctor's office when a tire on your car seems to be "going bad." Your doctor sends you to the emergency room for care, and your tire just "blows up." As you pull into the ER, a man who has witnessed this says: "I'll be glad to take care of the tire, sir; you just go get the care you need." And the patient gives the man his car key, to a total stranger. The car is a Mercedes Benz. The patient and his wife come in for care. He is refusing to put on a gown. He is very tense, but the nurse understands that Dialysis patients are some of the most difficult patients on earth. Did I mention he has cancer as well? The patient's needs were cared for. His wife confided to the nurse about the car. She said the man "looked like a military man." The nurse panicked a little inside and notified Security of her concerns. No one was that nice to strangers at night. The nurse asked what their faith was . . . in one unified voice; they said, "Christian." The nurse said: "Our God is an on-time God. You left this problem in God's hands, so let Him handle it. Angels come in many different forms, so a military angel works for me." She was so hopeful that God had sent a mechanically inclined angel to help. The nurse comes from a military family, and since Quantico was just an hour away, it could be a Good Samaritan helping. The patient spoke up and said, "We take military service as a moral responsibility; It means something." The nurse was hopeful but offered them a ride home if things didn't come to a positive end. The couple waited in the lobby, and no one came. They finally called the Sheriff's Department, and two deputies came to take a report. As I listened to the officers ask questions, I worried that I had been wrong to encourage this thinking . . . but I held out for a happy ending. About the time the story was done, a man came in holding a distinctive Mercedes Benz key and said: " I couldn't find one tire, so I put four used ones on your car. It pulls to the right, so you'd better get it checked." Everyone's mouth dropped. The officers were speechless. I put my arms around the wife as she dug in her purse for money. The Good Samaritan shook his head no and said, "You put that away. I didn't help you for the money, but the opportunity was my gift." The man came and took the wife's hand and said, "You holding my hand is all the thanks I need." We took the couple out to the car, and the wife asked what the plastic on the front seat floor was. I said, "That's what repair places do to keep your carpet clean." The wife broke down in tears again, "He really did it. We trusted him and he did the right thing!"

Now, the man still has cancer and still has to go to Dialysis, but he is back in charge of his life because a stranger cared. I believe in Angels. I saw one who had a retired military ID. I peeked over the shoulder of the Deputy and saw the man's name was Chris. Seems fitting and appropriate on November 11, 2021, Veterans Day.

6

Things people say . . .

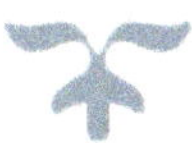

My husband went to pick up medicine at the grocery store pharmacy. Their pick-up window was closed, and the store appeared to be operating on less than their normal number of staff. He stood in line for forty-five minutes to get his meds and left. I noted on my phone that the price was $59. That was wrong, as the insurance had not been applied correctly, and I actively keep track of these things. Six phone calls later (they kept hanging up), I gave up, drove to the store, and got in the pharmacy line, starting out the front door in the parking lot. After sixty-three minutes, it was my turn. "NAME AND BIRTHDAY," the cashier screeched. I noticed her nametag said "Destiny," which struck me as funny.

I kept a calm tone and said, "Possibly, you should say hello and ask me what I want first. I believe you are the "technician" who shorted my kind husband $26.29." The nurse handed the sealed bag back to Destiny.

Destiny seemed annoyed. "I rang him up, and it's right, so take your medication. You don't know how busy we are. You people are just . . . (she hesitated) MEAN, and it's hard!" She started to tear up, and I noticed one of her elongated eyelashes had become partially unglued. It looked like her eyelid was suffering a stroke, but she kept on blinking.

I channeled my inner Julia Sugarbaker, from Designing Women, to reply to Miss Destiny. "Oh, I understand bad days better than you ever could. This is my second time standing in your line today because you wouldn't check the two insurances that are listed on the account. I am an ER nurse. I could do your job, my job, and CPR on the side and still look calm enough to have this conversation about why you won't give me my money back."

Destiny was determined and announced, "Well, you can't have it today; our manager isn't here." The wayward eyelash looked like it was trying to crawl away, but I didn't think offering a tissue was the right thing to do.

It was getting comical at this point. "OK, I'll take a Store Credit Card, cash, or you can sign an IOU, but I am not getting out of this line . . . not leaving the desk until I get my money." I noticed I had backup as the couple behind me began encouraging me with, "You go, girl!" Finally, Miss Destiny, the wayward cashier, brought me the money. The wayward eyelash was gone, but I noted the other one was hanging on for dear life. As I left, the customers behind me applauded.

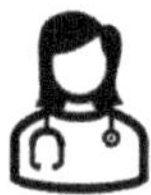

One of my nurse friends told me this: Her competitive six-year-old daughter has two older brothers. She came home from school and announced:

Daughter: "Noah kicked me in the balls."

Mom: "You don't have balls; only boys do, and we politely call them testicles," she said patiently.

Daughter: "When will I get some of my own?"

Mom: "Never . . . only boys have them."

Daughter: "It doesn't seem fair. Who fixes the problem? Is there a Saint I need to talk to?" (It helps to understand they are Catholic and have an established prayer order. Know that her mother is trying to look seriously concerned and trying desperately not to laugh at this point.)

Mom: "Well, it is probably best to ask God directly on that one. You could pray about it."

Daughter: "Do you think He will answer me?"

Mom: "If He doesn't, just add that to the list of things you need Him to address, and one day, give it to Him in person." Her daughter seemed happy with that.

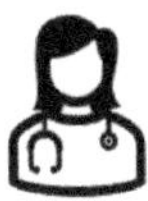

A "regular" patient was seen in the ER four times in one week for a very upset stomach. She misrepresented her earlier GI doctor's visit (they called ahead of her arrival at the ER).

Nurse: "The doctor wants me to start your IV and draw blood."

Patient: "OH GOD! I hope you have my narcotics in your pocket!"

Nurse: "No, ma'am. I have a limited amount of time that I can carry pain meds around, but after I draw your blood, I will get them."

Patient: (repeating louder and louder) "OH GOD! GOD! GOD make her do her job quickly. GOD! I'm dying!" If there were a drama queen award, we would give her the tiara.

Nurse: (in her most respectful voice) "So, ma'am, you're a religious woman?"

Patient: "What in the hell makes you think that?"

Nurse: "You keep calling out to God for help. Can I get you a Chaplain?"

Patient: "No . . . you can just do your job! I could use God to hurry you up about now!"

Nurse: "Well, He is sort of my boss, now that you bring it up. But if you yell at me and God, it just makes us nervous and slower . . . so you might want to consider that before you tell both of us off.

Patient: (opens mouth and closes it, content to just glare at me 'n God)

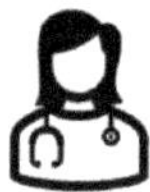

The Things People Say:

I find it odd that when people make stupid statements or ask inappropriate questions, they make it better by saying, "That's not really who I am as a person." Rarely do you hear, "I'm sorry. I am an idiot."

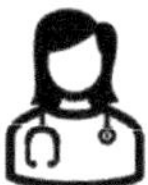

Today, I was referred to as "other non-physician staff." I'm not sure exactly what that means, but it didn't feel complementary. I double-checked my diploma, and it's not there either.

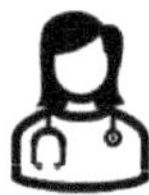

I saved a life today. I will never forget how good that feels. It's like your "fight song" on days when you're on the receiving end of poor patient satisfaction. I still have it!

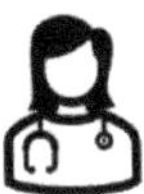

How do you define an ER nurse? "Adaptable, calm and collected during emergencies, quick-acting, big-picture thinkers, adrenaline junkies, lover of organized chaos, and their nursing shift report is something like "the patient is alive."

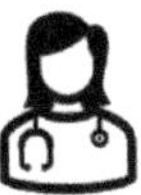

A nurse was questioning a doctor's orders, and the doctor said, "Do you see MD after my name? That means Makes Decisions." The nurse replied quickly, "Do you see RN after mine? It stands for Resists/Refuses Nonsense."

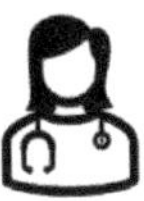

After a long night at work, as an ED nurse, it feels so good to come home and crawl into my own bed . . . but it feels even better to roll over and see my husband beside me with a shirt on that says PARAMEDIC. I can sleep in peace knowing I am well cared for.

7

Discernment in ways I will never understand

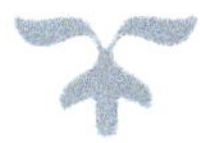

Sometimes, going to the lobby to get a patient is hard work. You get jumped by multiple people wanting to be seen now, and likely, the person you called for isn't answering. This time, the nurse went out through the ambulance bay and came back in the ER lobby door. She knew who she was looking for . . . she had an ID picture. The complaint? "I just don't feel like me." As the nurse approached the patient, the young woman made a dive through the crowd for the restroom. The nurse waited and waited a bit longer. Soon, the young woman came out of the Ladies' Room and said, "I'm here," but did not make eye contact. Realizing a familiar social awkwardness, the nurse invited her to walk outside and back through the ambulance bay to avoid the inevitable questions from the lobby crowd about why she got to go "first." She guided the patient to a quiet triage room. She seemed withdrawn but offered the nurse a handwritten note: "I have Asperger's Syndrome," which is a kind of autism. The nurse sat quietly and waited for her patient to speak first. That kind of introduction allowed the nurse to figure out that the young woman likely had a urinary tract infection (UTI) and was concerned about possible pregnancy from "a friend who isn't my friend anymore." She denied abuse. She had a UTI and was not pregnant. The nurse asked her to think of one person who loved her and wouldn't judge her to come pick her up. It took a while, but the young woman began to cry and said, "You." The nurse teared up, and the young woman hugged her until she couldn't hug anymore and abruptly pulled away. The nurse waited a few moments, wrote a checklist on her discharge papers, and gave it to the patient to review. She nodded affirmatively that she had cab fare home and could pay for her prescription. The nurse called her favorite cab driver and walked her to the taxi, giving the driver instructions (and an extra tip) to ensure medications were picked up and that the young woman got home safely. The nurse called her later to see if everything had gone according to plan, but the phone number was disconnected. To be completely alone, when you are surrounded by people, is so very difficult. Listen to others . . . you never know what they may be going through. And while you can't fix everything, you might make the walk a little easier for both of you.

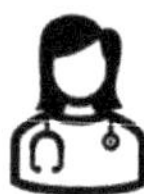

A call comes in to notify the staff that an officer is bringing a combative patient for medical clearance (she's going to jail). A thin, meth-head female in cuffs is brought in, complete with no shoes and bad language. The officer has the vest on with everything from taser to extra cuffs and leads the girl to the stretcher. He's tough and by the book, but the nurse notices he handles the patient carefully. Just before being arrested, she ran and was tackled by police who were checking themselves carefully to see if they were hit by the syringe and needle, she had in her hand. The process moves forward. The officer turns his back to the patient and asks the nurse if she can provide some kind of suitable clothing for the patient, so she won't have to wear the hooker outfit to be booked at the jail. He is also concerned she hasn't eaten in two days. His face is that of a caring father. The nurse is thinking of her family member, who is in the same spot. Both know they cannot change the inevitable, but at least for the moment, they can dress and feed her and make some preparation for the night to come and the long wait in jail. Social services show up to discover the whereabouts of her two-year-old daughter and find foster care at 3:00 a.m. in the morning . . . no easy task. The officer showed me her driver's license . . . she was beautiful at one time; now she has the masque of drugs and prostitution; she is no longer "mom"; she is detainee # 269475. The officer leads her out to his car. Another patient comes in with chest pain, and the nurse begins again.

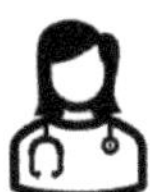

From a triage chair, you see a different side of the world. The nurse sees a man with his jeans around his knees, waiting to check-in.

Nurse: "Sir, I need to tell you, I think your jeans slipped down while you were waiting to be seen."

Patient: "I have underwear on, so what's the problem?"

Nurse: (trying to look old and somewhat feeble-minded) "Well, I can see you have underwear on, but you might not want everyone looking at it . . . and I can see your butt crack too. I'd hate for you to walk out and be embarrassed."

Patient's wife: "I told you so!"

Nurse: "I can give you a blanket to cover up with if you need it . . . we are here for you."

Patient: "You know nothing about fashion."

Nurse: "Maybe not, but I think only your wife should see you in your birthday suit."

Patient: (pulls up pants) "You all are just (he struggled to find the right word) . . . stupid."

Wife: "Well, stupid is as stupid does . . ." The phrase just hung there for a moment before his wife thanked me and walked out of the hospital. Eventually, the patient decided it just wasn't his day to be seen either.

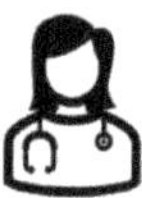

There was a moment when I thought I would stop breathing. Patients can become very chatty and treat the ER doctor like he is their personal family physician; it gets interesting. I was in the room when a doctor stopped the one-sided conversation to ask about the family history of an older woman with chest pain.

Doctor: "So, are your parents still living?"

Patient: (tearing up) "No, they are gone to their reward."

Doctor: "Can you tell me what your mother died from?" (patient hesitates and sniffles). "Was it a cardiac event?"

Patient: "No . . . she drowned." At this point, I thought we should just leave the room, but that reflex to ask questions just kicked in, and the doctor said . . .

Doctor: "And your father, did he have a cardiac event?" (Patient begins to bawl outright. I start handing out tissues.)

Patient: "No, I don't think he had a heart attack . . . He was with my mom." Thankfully, the doctor left . . . and I didn't have the heart to ask if her parents could swim.

8

Did I hear you correctly?

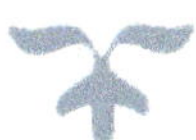

I couldn't post this at the time since I was already on the naughty list for some other meaningless infraction. Let me set the scene for you. It's night shift. Police brought in a middle-aged white male in overalls with no tee shirt, drunk, inappropriate, and loud, heading for a mental health room evaluation. I couldn't get near him. He kept screaming, "You ain't man enough." I considered an initial approach and put a plan together. I grabbed a Skoal can from a hidden shelf and dumped the contents in a trash can. After thoroughly washing the container, I dried it and bought two big Tootsie Rolls from the lobby vending machine. Using the secretary's pencil sharpener, I ground them to shreds and placed them in the reinvented Skoal can. Dropping the canned treat in my back pocket, I explained the ruse to our beloved psychiatric evaluator, Chris, who was immediately on board, and we walked into the patient's room. The patient starts winding up every curse word he knows until the nurse pulls out the Skoal can and puts a pinch in her mouth. The psych evaluator asks for a dip, and the patient stands in stunned silence for a moment.

"Dang, lady, you've done that good." For the first time, the patient smiled and asked, "Can I have some?"

The nurse smiles. "Maybe once we get the questions out of the way." Meanwhile, Chris is accurately spitting in a cup he brought. My aim was not so good, so I swallowed mine, and the patient became genuinely worried. We smiled, fessed up, and had a good laugh. The new Resident doctor was getting ready to come in. He was not a staff favorite because he was just too sure of himself and, frankly, annoying. The patient didn't like him but said he'd cooperate if we helped him punk the doc, so we set it up by giving the can to the patient, and I waited with him. In comes the Resident, spouting off questions, and the patient pulls out the can, taking a pinch, and offering it to me, saying, "Ladies first." I accepted it with a smile, and the patient held it out to the new Resident. I thought our doctor would throw up as he ran from the room. Chris and I retired from active "dipping" after that. The kind patient was a gentleman the rest of the night, and the Resident was mad that he couldn't fire a nurse, but hey, it's night shift, right?

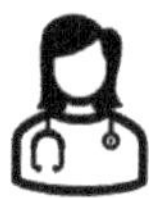

A patient came in with severe indigestion. The MD told the patient he probably had Barrett's Esophagus and gave him this explanation: "Barrett's esophagus or Barrett's oesophagus, sometimes called Barrett syndrome, Barrett esophagus, or columnar epithelium lined lower oesophagus (CELLO), refers to an abnormal change (metaplasia) in the cells of the lower portion of the esophagus. It is characterized by the replacement of the normal stratified squamous epithelium lining of the esophagus by simple columnar epithelium with goblet cells (which are usually found lower in the gastrointestinal tract). The medical significance of Barrett's esophagus is its strong association (about 0.5% per patient-year) with esophageal adenocarcinoma, a very often deadly cancer, because of which it is considered to be a premalignant condition." The patient said nothing, and the MD walked out.

Nurse: "Did you get that, or was it a little confusing?"

Patient: "I think so," but he looked worried. "Do I have cancer? And who is Barrett?"

Nurse: Realizing that the patient didn't get any of the confusing explanations, she strives to create a word picture of the problem. "Think of it this way. Your throat is all the people in Washington, DC. Your stomach is all the people in Georgia. When you eat something good, the people in Washington, DC, like it because they get the first taste, but the people in Georgia don't like being last in line, so they try to run and flatten the people in Washington, DC. Somewhere in the middle, the people of Virginia get pissed off and start fighting both sides. That is when you feel the acid in your throat."

Patient: "Oh, I get it." "It's sort of like a war between my stomach and my throat!"

Nurse: "You got it."

Patient: "So, who gets cancer?"

Nurse: "Mostly people who ignore the problem and don't get treatment. I'll give you instructions on who you need to follow up with to take good care of you."

Patient: "OK, but who is Barrett?"

Nurse: He's probably the MD's brother. You know how proud folks are of their families. The patient nodded, smiling, as he understood perfectly now.

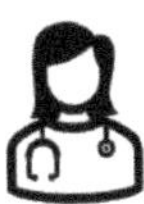

Once in a great while, nurses get a day off. On my day off, I decided to start planting our garden. Armed with potting soil, plants, seeds, and a wheelbarrow, I head to the storage area, only to be met by a honeycombed hornet' nest, actively being built. My better half was not home or available by phone. I went looking for some wasp killer spray, but of course, there was none to be found. I really needed to get my gardening tools. Every time I got near the door, they buzzed louder and flew larger rings around the hive. So, I found a bottle of super glue in my husband's wood shop. I've calmed patients down by singing before, so a song from Winnie the Pooh seemed appropriate, "It Looks Like Rain." I began singing softly and tip-toed near the hive, pouring super glue slowly on them, drop by drop. At first, it was no big deal and they kept working. However, as the flow of glue increased, they tried to fly at me. I backed up and noticed the hornet attackers losing altitude and sticking to wherever surface they landed on, permanently. Problem solved; gardening tools retrieved. But now I'm thinking about more practical applications at work . . . and I am smiling to myself.

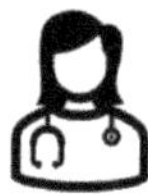

Wore my hair up in a braid on top of my head today. A sweet lady, who was used to speaking her mind, who was my first patient of the day.

"How pretty you are!"

I smiled and said, "Thank you so much. I don't get compliments often."

"It's nice, except for that Lizard on your head." I was speechless.

She took my hand and said, "But I love you, Lizard Lady."

I just smiled. "And I love you; doesn't everyone?" Lol.

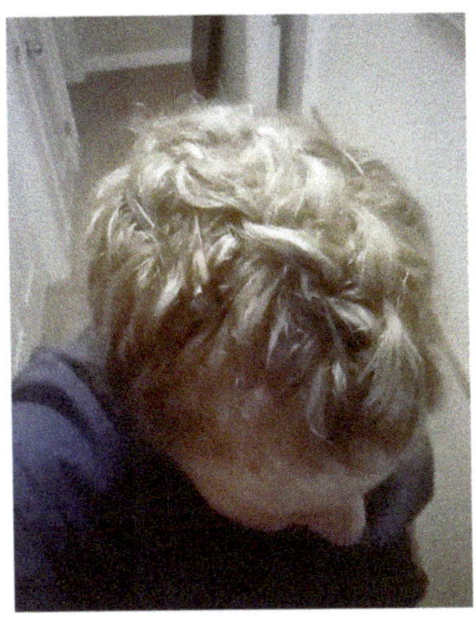

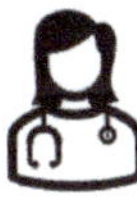

I've mentioned my student loans before. I called my loan company because I had been paying on them for ten years and thought that I was near the forgiveness date. I was trying to find out about student loan forgiveness after ten years of non-profit work. Sadly, I found out I had the wrong kind of loan. You cannot have Federal Loans-FFELP, only Direct Consolidated Loans for the ten-year forgiveness program to work, which no one kindly mentioned to me during the loan process. Here is the online transcript from the Navient Loan Program.

Kris Stegall: 10:30:26 a.m. I'm still looking for the correspondence and monthly statement part.

Adele B.: 10:32:52 a.m. Do you see the Get Correspondence Monthly Statements information?

Kris Stegall: 10:33:30 a.m. OK, I found it. Apparently, I am part of the wrong alphabet payment plan (FFELP) to qualify for the ten-year forgiveness program. It would be nice if someone had MENTIONED that to me. I am sixty-four and will be paying off my student loans with my retirement. So, I am not a fan of Navient.

You could have helped. Sallie Mae could have helped me, but you both chose not to.

Adele B.: 10:35:08 a.m. I'm sorry you feel that way. However, your loans are not eligible for the Public Service Loan Forgiveness program.

Kris Stegall: 10:38:00 a.m. Politically correct answer . . . but I have been an ER nurse at non-profit hospitals for my entire career. When I die, does Navient still get their cut? I'm planning and deciding how much insurance I need to carry, assuming I will still have to pay you off in death. Do you offer estate planning for this?

Adele B. 10:39:15 a.m. The Regulations governing your federal loans provide for forgiveness of an education loan in the cases of death. In order to ensure an account is serviced appropriately and to review loans for forgiveness, a copy of the borrower's death certificate would be needed. For more information on loan discharge due to death, you are welcome to visit StudentLoans.gov.

Kris Stegall: 10:40:27 a.m. OK, so if I die, I finally win? My family will be relieved. Thank you for your help

Adele B.: 10:41:09 a.m. You're very welcome. Live long and prosper.

She was doing so well up to that point. I paid off the loans and never regretted becoming a nurse. I do, however, regret my choice of career paths in obtaining my Master's in Nursing. I should have gotten better counseling and gone with Nurse Practioner, instead of Leadership. Leadership seemed very straightforward to me, but being a leader in professional nursing takes you completely away from the bedside, and that is what I love. I figured that if I knew all the ways the job could be done wrong, I'd have a leg up on doing it correctly. I am picture perfect in organizing care for massive disasters, but I didn't realize one of my first assignments would be figuring out how to back up the Titanic, find volunteers willing to be sacrificed, and pay everyone from the top down. Suffice it to say I went back to bedside nursing and have never regretted it.

9

Grace is a kindness given before you ask

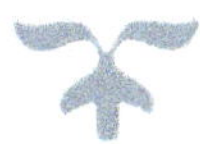

The nurse was taking care of an older patient who was slated to stay in the hospital but was stuck in the ER. Her son brought in beautiful flowers but couldn't stay because of family obligations. Things later changed, and the patient was going to be sent home. As she was being carried out in a wheelchair, she was holding the beautiful vase of roses. The patient noticed a young girl on a stretcher, under many blankets, not moving and struggling to breathe.

Patient: "Who's that? She looks sick."

Nurse: "She's my patient, and she is very sick. She is still sleeping off a procedure, but she may not live much longer."

Patient: (thinking out loud) "Nobody is with her . . . maybe she would like to wake up to some flowers. Nurse, can you give her these roses when she wakes up?"

Nurse: "Certainly can . . . I've never seen her get flowers."

Patient: Tears came to the woman's eyes. "Then just do it!" The lady was taken to her car, and the pink flowers were set on the counter near the young woman's stretcher.

At the end of her shift, half of the patients in the ER were waiting for a bed. The nurse's homicidal patient was acting out, the police were trying to control several situations, and the waiting room was overflowing. She gave a report on her patients to the incoming shift and then noticed the roses still sitting on the counter. Floral delivery was her next job. She took them upstairs to the young woman's room and other nurses on the patients' floor began asking, "Are those for Sue?" They were stunned and became visibly tearful when they heard the story of how a stranger cared. Sue was a chronic patient with no family and no visitors. Sue heard us, opened her sleepy eyes, and put a shaking finger over the end of her tracheostomy tube. There was a raspy whisper, but we all heard Sue say, "Thank You" and tears ran down her face. The Nurse thought you deserved to see what the power of a stranger who cares looks like.

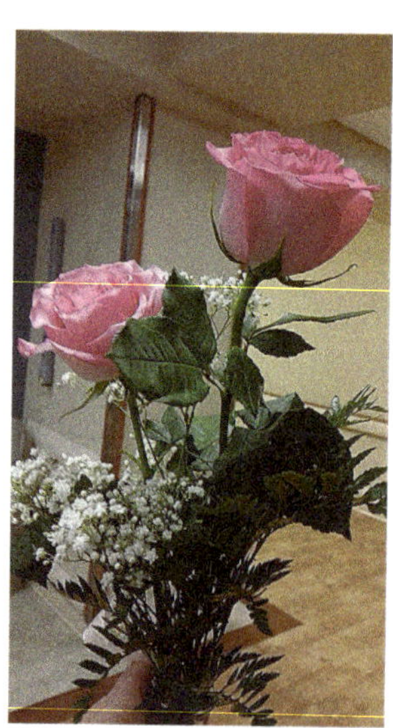

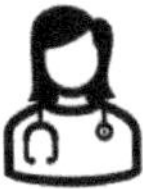

The nurse stood in a room with a patient today and listened to the doctor make mean remarks about the patient's management of her asthma. When the doctor turned his back to answer a phone call, the nurse reached out, took the patient's hand, and made a "quiet" gesture with a finger to her lips. She watched the tear fall onto the patient's gown and sat down beside her, giving her a tissue. The hurtful dialog continued . . . finally, the doctor left. The patient was going to leave without any treatment, but the nurse pointed out that the patient needed the medication that was ordered. At least the doctor had gotten that part right. The patient stayed and improved after a series of handheld nebulizers. The nurse later found the room empty, but that was no surprise. The nurse wondered if she had learned anything helpful about asthma management. Surely not, but the patient was schooled in the art of undiplomatic, passive/aggressive health care, and the nurse doubted she would see her again. The nurse spoke to the doctor afterward. Most ER docs treated her with respect and care. This doctor was kind enough to point out that she was not a doctor and unless she wanted to become a physician . . . well, the answer should be obvious. He turned back to his charting. ER nurses do not "dismiss" easily, so the nurse shared her career goal with the doctor. She aspired to be something more than just a doctor. She had always wanted to become a nurse . . . a good one. There was strained quiet, but the nurse patted his shoulder and said, "You'll get the hang of it," and she moved on to the next patient.

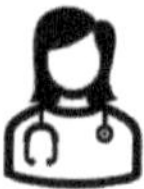

A funeral for a friend. Imagine, if you will, a funeral for a veteran in a small town called North Augusta, South Carolina. My knees knocked badly as I stood up in front of his friends and family to give the eulogy. He was the father I'd never had, but he stayed as close as I would let him, and I loved him for it. Mary Evelyn, his daughter and my best friend, rode behind the flag-draped coffin. As it traveled in the hearse, every car pulled over to the side . . . every police officer saluted . . ., and even people walking on the sidewalk stopped and snapped to a salute . . . young boys in camouflaged trucks not only stopped but took their ball caps off and put them over their heart, respectfully. Complete strangers were realizing the sacrifice and showing him the utmost respect. I was in the car behind that hearse last Sunday . . . and I saw what it meant to others, and I know what it meant to me. And it makes me sad that I don't see that more often.

10

Looking for the gift

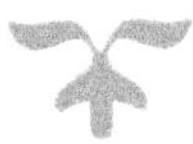

A friend's child passed away recently, and someone asked me how to know if they went to heaven . . . I remember the first time I saw a child die in an ER. Let me share it with you. An eleven-year-old was shot accidentally by his six-year-old brother. He was bleeding out, and his parents were rushing to get to the ER. A medical/admin/Police crowd gathered helplessly around the child, and the Doc ordered everyone out except a respiratory therapist, a paramedic, and me. Prepping him for surgery involved cutting his clothing off and establishing an IV. I told him his parents were coming and to hang on. He started sniffing the air and making chewing motions with his jaw . . . I thought he was going to seize. Then he said: "Don't you smell them? Um, fresh McDonald's Fries," and then, despite our best efforts, his heart stopped beating, and we could not restart it. A Paramedic alerted me that the parents had pulled up, and he would brief them on what their son would look like with a "'breathing tube" and all the tools we had at the bedside. He brought the parents in. They stood there in shock, taking the whole scene in. I stood a few feet away to give them grieving space but close enough to let them know why they couldn't touch their son. It was a Coroner's case due to the mechanism of death. After her initial tears, Mom asked me what his last words were. I was a little hesitant because I hadn't put the puzzle pieces together yet, but I told her. She started to laugh and cry at the same time. "He always said he knew the streets of Heaven were lined with McDonald's so angels could have French fries whenever they wanted them." The kid was on track . . . he just beat us there.

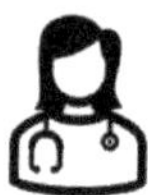

I was a new nurse trying to "talk" an IV into working at close range to a patient's left arm. My thick, curly hair, dark with blonde streaks in it and a loud touch of cinnamon (I'd dozed off in the stylist chair after a long night shift while getting my hair done). The patient was a lovely older Irish lady with a thick brogue who sounded delightful when she spoke. She was staring intently at my head during the process.

Patient: "You got that, now have ya'? I don't want to get needled again!"

Me: "Yes, I believe so. One more saline test, and I'll tape it in."

Patient: "Well, ya' know, my hair is gettin' thin on top, and I think I'll be getting me one of those wigs as you have. It's quite fetchin'."

Me: (sighing) "Well, I'd give you this one, but people would talk."

Patient: (Laughs, with that great Irish accent). "No, my darlin', I'll be gettin' my own wig! Maybe you should get another one, just in case ya' change your mind about the color."

Me: (note to self, never get your hair done the morning after you've worked all night)

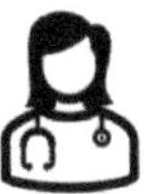

OK, the secret is out, and I am the envy of my nurse friends. I am going to hot yoga classes to try and regain some flexibility. The room is 105 degrees, and everyone's feet stink eventually. They say such nice things like "let go of whatever causes you pain or failure," and I'm sure they mean well, but what my mind hears is, "It's all about choices, so suck it up, buttercup and breathe it out, darlin'." They speak of working up to the "edge of your practice." I think this means I might need a "carry permit." My initial goal was to get through the hour without leaving, which I did. Now my goal is to do all the "downward dogs" without cheating. The instructor says we should look at our ankles with love and appreciate our neighbor's ankles as well. When I compare respective ankles, I find that mine have wrinkles and my neighbors do not. How does that happen? My knees feel a bit better, but the clincher for me to keep returning is the ice-cold, mint-scented washcloth they give out at the end. I swear it is as close to an ice-cold beer as I can get and still be able to drive. I think we should consider using the minty washcloths as part of the Advanced Cardiac Life Support protocol (ACLS governs how we save people). You could better resuscitate the dead if they knew that there was a prize involved. So, here's to hot yoga . . . just me, trying not to laugh out loud at the people who can imitate a human chair with their eyes closed, one foot raised . . . and not fall down. It's the prize I am after . . . the cool minty washcloth of success. We all gotta have a dream, right?

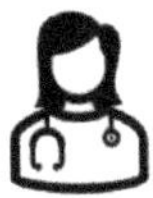

I just read a legal article on whether nurses should "hug" their patients . . . basically, it said you are safer, not hugging. I remember a seventy-six-year-old man who not only hugged me when he found out he was "cancer-free" but danced me out into the hall (he was wearing a hospital gown, no less) to show me his anesthesia had worn off completely. His wonderful wife asked me for the next dance . . . and we danced! We were all at the local church for the Wednesday night prayer meeting. When asked for prayer requests or answers, this sweet man announced to the church he was cancer-free and pointed me out as "his nurse." He walked over to my pew, offered his hand, and twirled me around twice. Everyone applauded! That was a proud and humble moment for me. Will there be hugs? Always. And will there be dancing? Definitely.

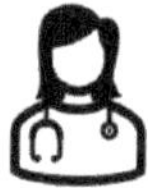

I volunteered to become a flight nurse in Columbia, South Carolina As an ER nurse, I was allowed to challenge the Paramedic test. It was a pre-hospital certification I needed if EMS didn't ride with us. I passed the test, and one of my first patients was an older man with a cardiac problem. In the middle of a diagnostic heart cath, the sheath (long tubing they use to thread tools into your heart's arteries) wouldn't move correctly. The patient needed to transfer to a full Cath lab, so Life Flight went to get him. I was by myself for this trip, but Chris, my pilot, was always ready to help in any way he could. We landed in the traffic circle of a small town. It looked a little like a celebration, with police cars aiming their lights at our landing area, but the transfer from EMS was made quickly. The patient, "Glen," was awake and in no pain but had a jumpy heart rhythm. He would take deep breaths occasionally and cough.

I didn't realize until we were up in the air that the heart Cath stent had been left in place. Sometimes, especially with patient movement, the heart stent will become irritating to the heart, like a place you wish you could scratch, but can't reach. I had no advanced training in this, so I checked with my ER doc and got permission to pull back just a bit on the stent, and it stopped the intermittent bad heart rhythm. Now we had about a twenty-five-minute ride home when our pilot said:

Chris: "If you look to the left side of the aircraft, you can see Halley's Comet coming over the horizon." That's a one-time, every hundred-year event. The patient wanted to see it but could barely hear our conversation. Chris handed the patient a set of headphones, and Glen and I watched the comet for about ten minutes. We knew people were expecting us at a certain time, and both Chris and I could be fired for "sight-seeing." I explained to Glen that while we could just say the trip took a bit longer, he could never tell anyone what we had witnessed since I would likely lose my job.

Glen: "How long do I have to keep my mouth shut?"

Nurse: "At least five years. I will have moved on by then."

Glen: "Well, that's okay. They don't think I will live more than two," he laughed. He smiled and was sworn to secrecy.

We landed, and Glen was whisked off to the Cath Lab. About two days later, I saw him being wheeled by on a stretcher. He put his hands up to his face like he was holding binoculars and then gave me a thumbs-up. It just doesn't get much better than that.

11

Does it pass the common sense test?

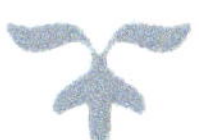

Things are never quite what they seem and getting patients to be honest takes patience.

Nurse: She begins taking notes and says, "So, can you tell me what happened?" (Two brothers lying side by side on separate stretchers, involved in the same incident. One with his nose broken and a possibly fractured jaw, and the other missing an ear, but the bleeding was controlled with a pressure dressing.)

Brother #1: Well, Ma'am, I was layin' in my own bed, mindin' my own business, when all of a sudden, there was a ruckus set in, and the next thing I remembered was when someone threw a TV set in my face." (The nurse keeps taking notes and nods at the second patient to tell his story.)

Brother #2: "Well, I was visitin' John tonight, and I got tired, so I lay down. Now I didn't hear nothin'." I'd gone to bed early, and I woke up with a big ole Ax beside my head . . . that sucker cut my ear off. Can it be put back on?" He hands her a tissue containing a skin flap, which she passes off to a technician to secure properly. She gets ready to sum up the story, like Sargent Joe Friday, from Dragnet.

Nurse: "OK, boys, let me see if I got this right . . . you and your buddy John here were perfect angels tonight and went to bed early, like choir boys getting ready for Church on Sunday. You bothered no one, never thought of stealing a TV, and don't remember seeing anyone who assaulted you. (Both men nodded, and the nurse, who was joined by a local Sheriff Officer, continued) Okey Dokey! Boys, I'm going to leave you to discuss this amongst yourselves because I have a bet going on with your Doctor that if I give you a little more time, you'll start to remember you were initially sitting on the front porch, sipping liquored-up sweet tea and telling respectful stories about your Moms, when some horrible man came by and asked you to drive the getaway car. You two angels, of course, refused to participate and went to bed early. That's why you forgot to lock your door and got the crap beat out of you. I'm betting you do not even have a night light, so you couldn't see the man's face.

Brother #1 and Brother #2: Yes Ma'am. Yes! It's like you were there.

Nurse: Somebody owes me dinner. (She hands her notes to the Sheriff and goes into the next trauma room.)

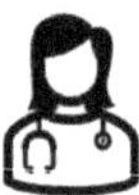

The nurse was watching *Maleficent*, starring Angelina Jolie, on a tablet during her lunch break. A wonderful EVS guy named Joseph stood behind her, staring at the movie. He was from Nigeria and had six children so the nurse felt he might know the movie. Joseph shook his head "no."

Joseph: "It is a very grown-up movie, I think," shaking his head sadly.

Nurse: "It's a fairy tale for children and families. It has fairies and a happy ending."

Joseph: (pointing to the screen) "What is this "fairies?" So, the nurse tries to describe fairies as mythical creatures who do good things.

Joseph: Points to Angelina Jolie and proclaims loudly, "That is a flying bat. I bet she has long toenails and hangs upside down at night . . . she has big wings like a bat." Joseph is flapping his arms for emphasis now. "She is killing the army using walking trees." Now he is stomping around the room. "It is too scary for my children." Then he wonders aloud, "Is she the fairy who steals the children's teeth?"

Nurse: "She's not a bat. She doesn't steal teeth. She's a fairy and saves the day at the end of the movie."

Joseph: "Why does she not start now? She could do a lot of good things faster. I do not think she is a good fairy . . . not like your Santa Claus!"

Nurse: She exhales and smiles at Joseph. "Maybe we should start doing good things now," and closed the movie.

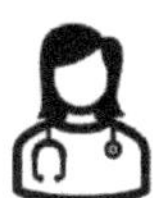

I didn't write about this at the time, but I think it might be useful, especially to student nurses. I was a student nurse working as a float technician on the night shift in a Women's Hospital. Assigned to an orthopedic floor, I felt comfortable and began making my rounds (we didn't get a formal report but checked with the nurses later). One of the first rooms I went in had a young female covered in sweat but breathing and groaning. I pulled the blood-soaked sheet back to find a tiny infant, slightly blue, about two pounds, intermittently gasping for air. The patient could speak, had no external monitoring, and seemed oriented. I put her nurse light on, wrapped the baby in a towel, and ran to the nurse's station.

Me: "The lady in room 302 just delivered this in her bed. It's female, with respirations of about ten, no crying, and limp muscle tone."

Staff: "Just hand it to me," said a charge nurse, so I did.

Me: "What should I do now?"

Staff: "Just check on all your other patients; I will take care of her."

So, I did. Near the end of my twelve-hour shift, I noticed the young lady dressed and escorted out in a wheelchair. I found out that her baby had simply been placed in a storage area to die alone. At the end of my shift, I went down to the VP of Nursing. I knew her to be a fair and nonjudgmental Nurse. I explained what happened and asked why the patient wasn't on the maternity floor.

VP: "We don't like to mix "evacuations" and the joy of new births for several reasons, but you should not have been involved with this patient. I'm sorry you were introduced to the process this way."

Me: "I am a student and do not wish to make a formal complaint. I will willingly take care of patients who have had abortions for any reason, but I do not want to be part of the team that initiates the process unless the infant has died or the mother is in immediate danger of dying. Would the hospital accommodate that?"

VP: "We will do our best, within reason. If it comes up, please contact the charge nurse or house supervisor. But tell me, what was your biggest concern with this process?"

Me: I thought for a moment and said, "The baby was gasping for breath, and even though I was pretty certain it wouldn't live, I thought someone should take the time to hold and comfort the child as it died."

There was a thoughtful look on the VP's face, and she agreed.

Fast forward to my ER/NICU days: If a baby was born less than 500 grams (just a tad over a pound), no lifesaving efforts were made. Gill slits, webbed fingers, and fused eyelids were warning signs that the baby was too premature to live. But on my watch, not one baby died alone. Nurses were eager to wrap them in warm blankets and rock them if the parents couldn't. I went on to have three miscarriages and a stillborn son at seven months, so I do have an idea of what mothers go through, be it elective or non-elective terminations to pregnancy. I've stayed away from most of the political frays on women's rights but feel that a woman and her care provider should make these decisions based on healthcare and personal beliefs. It's not about judging but about caring. I hope that sharing my experience will help a new nurse figure out her caring path.

12

Who is in charge here?

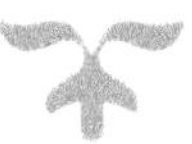

I have a wonderful friend, Chris, who is the "psych-guy" (code for intake evaluator) who assesses our mental health-challenged patients. He sent me this story from my old ER, and it's priceless.

It is early Christmas morning, and the night shift is getting ready for shift change. Two officers are dragging a woman singing at the top of her lungs. "Smoking crack and sniffing glue. Smoking crack since I was two." Our beloved psych-guy was in the ER, finishing up paperwork. The songstress had no psychosis or delusions but was as high as a kite. Staff agreed to "metabolize her to freedom", which is code for releasing her home when she is ready so she can be with her kids on Christmas.

Psych-guy: "How much crack have you smoked?"

Patient: "5 cents" and laughs.

Psych-guy: "You can't smoke 5 cents. Maybe $50 worth, and you'd be on the other side of the ER and probably dead. Listen, we're trying to get you home to be with your kids for Christmas, where you belong . . .. Not here or in jail."

She finally starts answering questions. Intake talks to the doctor and orders some meds, so with a plan in place, she can finally go home. We allow her to make a few calls, and the family agrees to pick her up when she is ready.

Another combative patient comes in, and we move the crack-smoking woman to a chair in the hall to wait for her family. The Trauma nurses are now singing Christmas carols over the intercom. The crack-smoker joins in the singing, and the woman has quite a set of pipes. It's almost beautiful, and *she knows the words*! She's manageable now that she has a "job," so we let her go down to Trauma and sing Christmas carols until her ride picks her up. The effect was calming. Christmas morning with our medical family. I love my work family. Holidays with them are always enjoyable, especially in my tired state of mind.

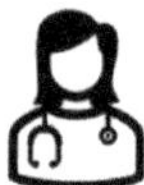

A "physician" came storming through the ER, loudly complaining that a "nurse didn't know what her job was . . . why was she even here?" He continues to complain that she simply runs away from her "duties." The staff nurse heard the doctor complaining and told him he "could not yell in this department." Then she politely asked, "How may I help you?" The doctor, a "water-walking" specialist, said he could do whatever he wanted to do. The nurse stood up, with only a counter in between them.

Nurse: "You can be angry, mad, irritated, enraged, pissed off, and unhappy, but you cannot announce it within earshot of patients; not in this department." The specialist stormed up and pounded his fist on the nurse's counter right in front of her. The ER Doctor moved in between the angry nurse and the charging doctor.

ER Doc: Turning towards the nurse, he said, "Just put some oxygen on the patient . . . I'll take care of it." The specialist exhaled loudly and stormed off.

Nurse: (to ER Doc, who was known to be a little hard for staff to manage) "Ya' know, if anyone ever said you were a jerk to staff, they'd be wrong because you don't hold a candle to that sad excuse for a doctor. If he were on fire, he'd be lucky to have someone spit on him."

ER Doc: He smiled for the first time and said, "So, you'd at least spit on me?"

Nurse: "Absolutely . . . we all would!"

ER Doc: "I'm starting to like it more and more around here," and he walked off smiling.

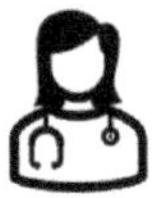

If you can make a word picture of the problem, parents understand it better. A mom brought the youngest of their brood to the ER with "trouble breathing." Usually, these children have a history of respiratory problems.

Me: "Mom, do you smoke?"

Mom: "Yes, but we never smoke in the same room as him."

Me: OK, let's take that thought process one step further. If we are in a pool together, is it okay if I swim to the other side and take a poop? (stunned silence from a chatty Mom as she thinks about exactly what that means)

It's amazing to see that people still have "lightbulb" moments.

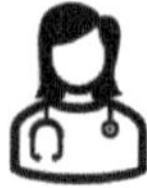

A little girl comes to the ER with an upset stomach. One dose of over-the-counter anti-nausea medication and no more vomiting! The Dad thinks more tests should be run because if it were *that* easy to fix, he'd have stayed home . . . hmm.

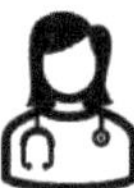

We transport patients almost everywhere because it's faster, and they don't get lost or change their minds about getting a test.

Cranky Patient: "I don't want to ride in the wheelchair; I'll look like a patient."

Nurse: "Not if I drive." (The nurse wheels the patient extra fast to get through both sets of automatically closing doors at the same time, barely making it.)

Patient: "What the hell? This is like a bad rodeo."

Nurse: "Hey, it gets better. We're going to CT scan next. We can wear cowboy hats and take the stairs!"

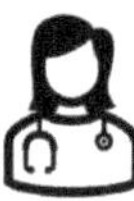

I actually took classes in Disaster Medicine, so I could identify when to pull the disaster trigger. The rest becomes an algorithm when they declare the day an official disaster, and it becomes a simple, more direct approach to emergency care. Assign people to four groups . . . The minor group just goes home to nurse their boo-boos. The delayed group gets snacks and takes turns telling each other how they got hurt. The immediate group gets curbside service, and the last group eventually goes "home to heaven'" in a few minutes or goes to surgery. It's a simple map that everyone can follow. But if it's not an official disaster, you may still feel exhausted halfway through the day, but you must control your "inner voice." A verbal filter is helpful, and the ability to say, "I'm *so* sorry your expectations did not meet your observations," without choking, is a real bonus. (I learned that line when I was made to formally apologize to a physician when I had done the right thing.) The outcomes are eventually the same, but at least with a Disaster, there are directions, assigned resources, and destination tags for patients. Regular bad days come with the drive-thru mentality that just says, "I want it my way immediately. I want your manager's name and the CEO's phone number, now!" If we stand there staring off for a moment, give us time to try and engage our verbal "filter." We probably haven't peed or eaten in hours, creating low brain sugar and a high blood pressure circle of repetitive thinking. Chances are good that whatever we say will not fix things. Before either of us says something that we cannot walk back, take a breath. Hug a nurse, feed EMS, run interference for those who are not able to rise to the occasion, don't yell at the doctor, and do not fake chest pain, thinking you will get to be "first." We take that seriously and there will be tests forthcoming. We love our jobs, no matter how challenging they may be, and have chosen to be here for you (They don't let us accept monetary tips either). Emergency care . . . use it wisely.

13

Love never fails

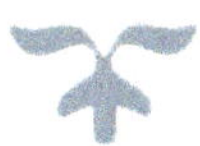

An ER nurse was fifteen minutes away from finishing a very long twelve hours. Trying to help (at 3:00 a.m.), she volunteered to take the hypertensive dementia patient to her room. Going up the elevator, the nurse had to sit on the stretcher with the patient to keep her from jumping off. As they traveled down a silent hallway, the nurse gently said, "Better be quiet, or you'll wake the babies." Instantly, the patient lowered her voice, and the nurse delivered her to the room. The patient wouldn't get into bed until she had inspected every piece of furniture and flushed the toilet four times. Finally, the nurse steered the empty stretcher down the hall toward the elevator so she could head home. She noticed a tiny little woman waving her down from a well-supported hospital bed. The woman was frail and lost among the mountain of pillows that held her in place. The nurse parked the stretcher and went into the woman's room. (The administration doesn't want us to do this because we know nothing about the patient's care.) She noted that there were three IV pumps keeping blood pressure and heart rate controlled and that the woman's delicate face was padded so that the high-pressure oxygen tubing would stay in place.

Nurse: "I'm Kris . . . what can I do for you?"

Janell: "I'm Janell. Take me home or send me home."

Nurse: (noticed her purple DNR bracelet) "Do you want to go to your home, or are we talking about going home to heaven?"

Janell: "Either one, as long as I get to hug my gran'babies one more time." Tears welled up in Janell's eyes, and Kris leaned over the bed, only to have the bed alarm go off! So, she pulled up a chair and held Janell's hand.

Nurse: "I wish I could, but I can't. What else can I do for you?"

Janell: "Come closer." The patient strained to get past all the monitoring equipment and IV lines to kiss the nurse's cheek. With a tear falling down her cheek, Ms. Janell told the nurse to have a good night and thanked her for stopping to check on her. The nurse kissed her back and left to take the empty stretcher back to the ER. The nurse's heart was officially broken by the kindness of a grandmother's tears.

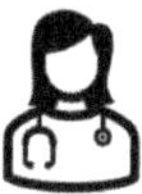

At some point in time, we all face the death of a loved one, or as a nurse, it may be a stranger who has no family. There are names given to people left behind after a death. A wife who loses her husband becomes a widow. A husband who loses his wife is a widower. A child who loses his parents becomes an orphan. But parents who lose a child face a vast and sudden emptiness. It is said that when a parent dies, you feel like you've lost your past, but when a child dies, you feel as if you've lost your future. My resolve is to take a leap of faith, believing without the benefit of proof, and learning to see with my soul and listen with my heart. Grief and pain are something you hold inside, and they become part of your DNA. The temptation is to never speak of the pain again, but only in feeling the sadness, can we become open to the lesson it teaches and nurture the inner healing. You never forget, but you resume the journey. I believe hearts are broken so that they remain open to remember the truly important things; I believe in the love . . . it bears all things, believes all things, hopes all things, and endures all things. Love never ends . . . and I am so glad for that!

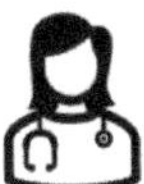

Janice, an older woman, had been in hospice care for over a year. Her family couldn't come to terms with her dying at home, and she didn't want to stay in an end-of-life facility, so every time her health failed, she came to the ER. This time, she looked pale and was having trouble breathing. After completing the triage and initial nursing care, I went to brief the doctor on what we had done in the past. She would be admitted. There were only supposed to be two visitors at one time, but crowds never scared me, so I overlooked the rule and simply kept the curtains closed. I went back into the room to apply oxygen and noticed four family members lined up on a wall. I finished my duties and sat on the edge of the bed to speak to Janice at eye level. I wear hearing aids, but I occasionally miss things, and it appeared everyone was listening to something. Janice motioned for me to stand up, and I did. One of the family members saw my confusion and said, "You were sitting on top of Aunt Bell." They motioned me to sit at the foot of the bed. I moved as directed and kept silent, waiting to better understand the dynamics in the room. Janice spoke up and said, "Aunt Bell thinks you are one of the nicest nurses she's ever met."

"Thank you very much. I've not had a compliment like that in a long time. Which of you is Aunt Bell?" I asked. Janice said that

Aunt Bell had died a number of years ago, and she always showed up when a family member was going to die. She motioned to the place where I had been initially sitting. I just nodded. Everyone in the room seemed at peace with this process, and I felt valued to be included. I asked Janice if she was going to die tonight. The entire family shook their head no, and Janice said Aunt Bell told her it wasn't time yet. I was good with that. I excused myself and called a report to the receiving medical floor. To my surprise, they knew about Aunt Bell and were satisfied that Janice would make it through the night. It gave me a warm fuzzy feeling to be included in that kind of love.

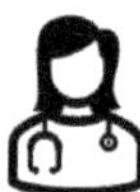

It's been a challenging week, but when I look at the team I work with, I have no doubts I am in the right place at the right time. It's rare to know you are exactly where you should be . . . I am . . . and if I forget, even for a moment, I am surrounded by those who remind me. Thank you so very much.

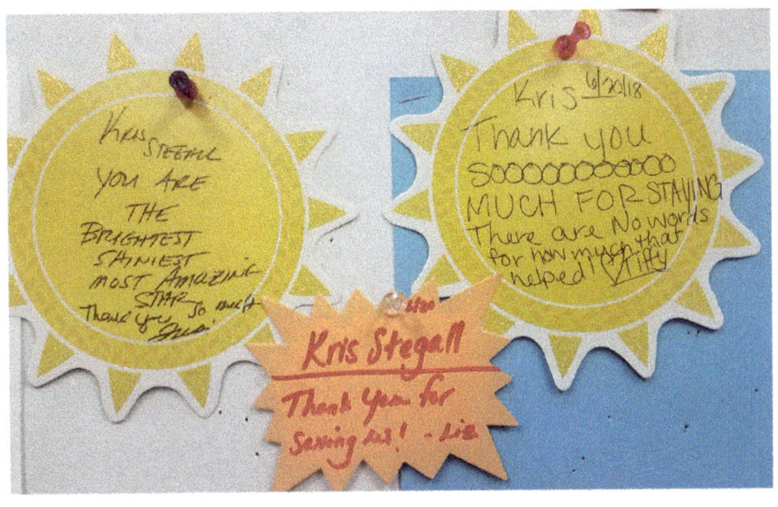
KRIS STEGALL
YOU ARE
THE
BRIGHTEST
SHINIEST
MOST AMAZING
STAR
Thank you so much
Kris 6/20/18
Thank you
SOOOOOOOOOOO
MUCH FOR STAYING
There are No words
for how much that
helped! ♡ Tiffy
Kris Stegall
Thank you for
Saving us! - Liz

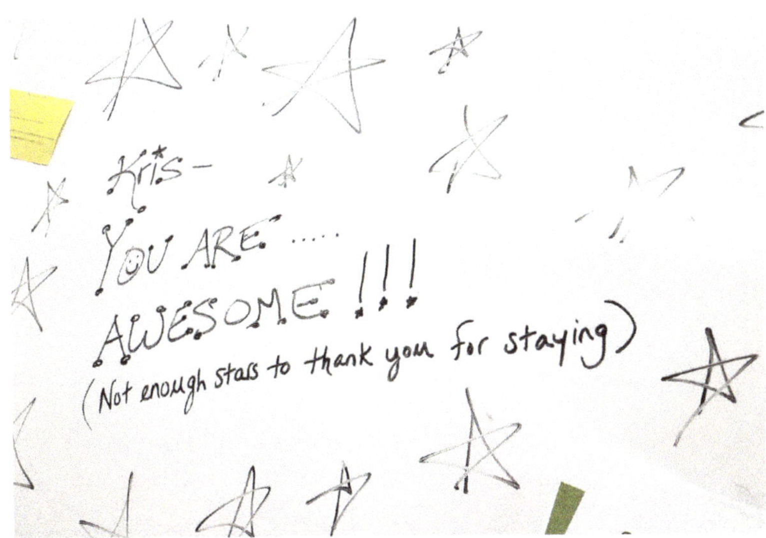
Kris-
YOU ARE .....
AWESOME!!!
(Not enough stars to thank you for staying)

14

We all have a job

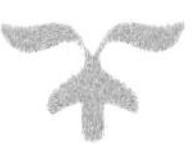

It was a snowy night in Virginia. Big snowflakes were lighting up the sky, and the hospital ER entrance was a bit icy. A family of four was escorting a member home. One of the unruly kids was nine years old and had ADHD. He'd missed his meds today and was all over the place. Dad tried to keep him in check but had to leave to get the car. I was the adult in charge and escorted them all to the discharge area. The fast-moving boy saw the snow and ran out into it, not looking for cars, falling and getting back up repeatedly. As the family put their injured person into the car, I noticed Dad opening the back door and calling to his son. I don't know what possessed me, but I picked up two handfuls of snow and launched them in the kids' direction. Now he had a challenge. I grabbed another nurse to help, and we pounded him with snowballs unmercifully. At first, Dad was angry, but when the kid didn't respond to his shouted directions, a smirk crossed his face, and he picked up a snowball and threw it at his rowdy son. The kid was overwhelmed and ran for the safety of the car. Dad smiled and said thanks before driving away. Oh, the joys of being a discharge nurse on a snowy night!

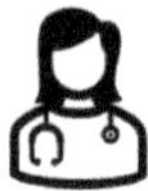

Dear Administration: With the extra patient loads you've given us; we have developed a working plan for handling the frequent call lights. We've given several confused, long-term patients your name and title and told them to yell for you if they need anything. We feel confident that by working together, we can keep the Press Ganey Scores up.

Team Love,
The Nurses

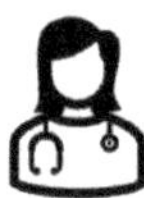

It was a long day, and traffic was slow on the way home. The tired nurse was intent on stopping by the local fast-food establishment to grab dinner. She waited her turn at the speaker to order.

Nurse: "Two famous bowls, please."

Speaker Voice: "Would that be all?"

Nurse: "You got a suggestion?"

Speaker Voice: "Why yes, I do. How about a Sauvignon Blanc and a side order of Calamari?"

Nurse: "I think I'm in love!"

Speaker Voice: "Had a long day? We are here for you, ma'am!"

Nurse: "I'll definitely be back."

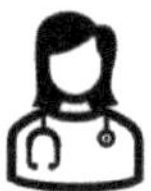

I took out student loans to pay for my nursing education. Let me know when we get to the part where someone else will pay off $10,000 of my student loans. I may not have really understood the terms of the agreement when I initiated the paperwork for the money, but I owned them for over twenty-five years and paid them off. It was my job, my honor, and my privilege to complete the agreement. I earned my degree; no one gave it to me. I fought tooth and toenail, worked multiple jobs, and managed a family. So, if everyone gets to go to school for free and gets their loans paid off, will everyone be happy? (Not if my taxes go up . . .) I think that we may be seeing fewer nurses who are competent to perform the complexities of the job or are willing to work weird hours and holidays. Did I mention that? We all work a minimum of three major holidays a year, take call and work weekends. Your Paid Time Off can be canceled if the unit cannot be "adequately" staffed. It's not for the faint of heart. Why would anyone want to be a nurse? For me, it's the hugs, humility, and grace that others show me as they die. It's the ability to save lives, give second chances, hold the hand of a frightened child and give them teddy bears-books-and homemade blankies, or be the person to brush grandma's hair fifty strokes in the morning and hand her clean dentures so she can speak clearly. You haven't lived until you walk the sweet dementia woman down the hall so she can throw socks at people she doesn't like. Frankly, if you don't have the heart for nursing, find another line of work. So, if it's not your cup of tea, don't take out the loan. If you do choose a profession where a loan is necessary, make sure you understand the repayment terms.

15

Holidays in the ER

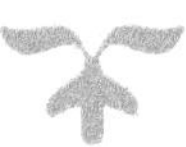

It was an air freshener kind of night. It was one of those nights that made me want to share the active state of urgency with staff, patients, and total strangers. It was Christmas Eve, and everyone wanted to be home before midnight. I believe the Charge Nurse was determined to sort out all the roadblocks and kick common sense into high gear. Many admitted patients had rooms, but there was always a reason why they couldn't go there. Lost time was the shared enemy. She gathered all the Situation, Background, Assessment, and Recommendation (SBAR) reports on admitted patients, faxed them to the appropriate floors, waited fifteen minutes, and called the receiving nurses to transport their ER patients. This caused some grumbling in the ranks, but after giving and cleaning up after two huge enemas, being spit on with precise accuracy that only an eight-year-old wearing a Batman shirt could pull off, running from a wheelchair speed racer and cleaning the vomit off two unsuspecting police officers, we were not looking to win awards. Our salvation came in the form of Ocean Breeze air spray! The hospital did not allow us to have it but it's always in somebody's locker. Heaven knows how many banks we could hold up if we each had a sprayer, but now we could take a deep breath without waiting to pass out. Things settled down, and then SHE came in. A sweet graceful young woman, not demanding our help but asking for it.

Young Woman: "I can't breathe so good because I got twenty-seven tumors on my liver, and now, they've had babies. They've started to take over my lungs." She coughed and cleared her throat. "I just came into town to be with my mom this Christmas." The staff seated her in the open Trauma Bay and started the triage process.

Nurse: "It must be a special Christmas." Her blood pressure was 95/52, a bit low, the nurse thought. Her skin was cool and dry but very pale.

Young Woman: "Yes, and probably my last," she added haltingly, in almost a whisper "I need to tell her I stopped the chemo because it doesn't help anymore."

Nurse: "I bet she cries." The nurse sat down beside her and held the young girl's hand as tears slipped down her face. Suddenly she felt humbled and grateful. Staff was aware of the young woman's concerns, and things began to appear on her stretcher as if by magic. We had a casual conversation during her initial care and heard there was an eleven-year-old brother. A gaily wrapped package was placed on her stretcher labeled "my brother." Her mom liked shiny hair gel, so the next wrapped package had a "Mom" tag on it. One nurse gave up her Christmas meal so that the patient could have a proper dinner. We kept her for Observation, planning to take her home in the morning, hoping to be able to make this Christmas special. The end of the shift was Christmas morning, and staff had families to get home to, but three of the staff made it their goal to take the patient "home" to keep from sending her off in a cab. They literally fought over who would escort the patient home. In the end, they all rode together. After all, this will be the last Christmas with her family.

Now what would you do if that was your story, and you knew what the ending would be? I went home and hugged my family.

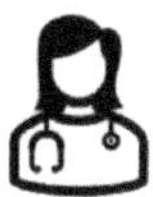

The ER nurse, is jokingly called a jack of all trades and master of none, is often floated to work on different units. Tonight, it was the adult ICU. Her first patient was a young female who had a cocaine overdose, was being managed on multiple IV medications, and was currently intubated on a ventilator. An older couple walked in during the initial assessment. The nurse knew that the ICU generally made the family wait until they had reviewed the patient and doctor's orders, but it didn't seem worthwhile to chase out the family tonight. ER Nurses are used to working in front of a crowd. The gentleman introduced himself as "Granddad." His first question asked was directed to care in the ER.

Grandfather: "Didn't I see you downstairs tonight? You work in the ER, right?" The nurse kept busy giving medications but nodded yes. "I thought you looked familiar. You took care of us two weeks ago when we came to the ER. Do you remember us?"

Nurse: (smiles) "Yes, I do, but a few stitches took care of things last time. This is a lot different." They watched the cardiac monitor run through its paces and heard the rhythmic click every time their granddaughter's chest rose as air jiggled the tube that "breathed" for her.

Grandfather: "It doesn't matter why we had to come back, 'cause you cared for us. We needed help, and you showed us how we could get it. Now, we need a little more, and you are still here. When we came in the first time, you fixed us up just fine. I remember when we were discharged, you took the time to walk us to the lobby. You hugged each of us, and it made us "tear up" to think that a stranger would care that much about an older couple. Now you're taking care of our precious granddaughter."

Nurse: (taking their hands) "Sir, it is rare that anyone tells me something like that. You've made me feel so very special to be a nurse, your nurse. You've made my day."

She reached over and squeezed the patient's hand and felt a slight squeeze back . . .

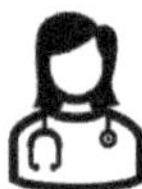

It turned out to be the best Halloween I'd had in years. An elderly woman arrived for a psychiatric exam. She has been "acting out," and her family was no longer able to care for her, so they called the Police, who delivered her to the ER for evaluation. The standard protocol is to get the patient in a gown and remove all personal belongings. The nurse enters the room about the time the patient has put on a gown but is hanging on to her "snapper" purse for dear life. Nothing else seems to matter. The nurse calls for a quiet moment and sits down on the bed beside the woman, who has her purse tucked under her gown.

Nurse: "Hi, I'm your nurse today. Could you tell me what's in your purse?"

Patient: "You wouldn't understand. I must take care of her. You won't do it."

Nurse: In a softer voice and touching the woman's arm. "Take care of who?"

Patient: "You'll think I'm crazy."

Nurse: "Maybe not. You'd be surprised by what I believe. What's in your purse?"

Patient: "No! You'll not take care of her!" pulling the purse away. Hoping to prevent a fight, the nurse waves Security off for a few more moments.

Nurse: "I can keep a secret . . . is she in your purse?"

Patient: "Yes . . . she's my fairy princess, and I have to take care of her."

Nurse: "Can I see her? I'll be quiet so I won't frighten her."

Patient: The patient looks both ways to make sure it is safe. The nurse mimics her motions, looking both ways, and nods approvingly. The patient starts to open her purse. "Be *really* quiet because she spooks *really* easy . . . she's nervous around new people." (She carefully opens the purse and then closes it quickly.) The patient is smiling at me for the first time. "Isn't she beautiful?"

Nurse: "She's the prettiest fairy I've seen all day . . . Is she yours?" (Noting the empty purse, the nurse elects to let the patient hold on to it).

Patient: "Yes, and I am responsible for her. I need to keep her with me."

Nurse: "I understand now. Think she might be hungry?"

Patient: Smiling now, "Oh yes, some apple juice and graham crackers would be lovely for her."

Nurse: "I think I have enough for the two of you." The lady is calmer now, knowing she can keep her pocketbook. After all, we all have special things we hold on to just to get through the day. We could all use an extra fairy princess some days!

Epilogue

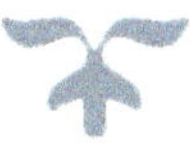

The daily life of ER nursing is never routine and has filled my life with new "presents" to open every day. I wouldn't trade the life I've had for anything in the world. Thank you for sharing some of these moments, from the heart of an ER nurse, with me.

www.ingramcontent.com/pod-product-compliance
Ingram Content Group UK Ltd.
Pitfield, Milton Keynes, MK11 3LW, UK
UKHW062257290726
14090UKWH00017B/743

9 798868 506086